advance praise for

The Boy Who Could Run But Not Walk

"This book is chock-full of cases of children with cerebral palsy who vastly exceed their physicians' expectations, as well as practical advice for parents and caregivers on how this can be done. Karen Pape, MD, is a pioneer, rightly demanding that colleagues integrate the new science of brain plasticity as it applies to these children, and this is her *cri de coeur*, recording not only the new breakthroughs, but effectively explaining why, tragically, so many families are still denied these important interventions."

—*Norman Doidge, MD, author of* The Brain's Way of Healing *and* The Brain That Changes Itself

"Full of wisdom, deep scientific and medical understanding, wonderful practical advice, and justified hope."

—*Michael Merzenich, PhD Professor Emeritus, UCSF, author of* Soft-Wired, *and winner of the 2016 Kavli Prize for Neuroscience*

"An affirmation of the life-changing benefits of neuroplastic healing and some powerful lessons for life."

—*Jay Greenspan, MD, MBA, Neonatologist, Pediatrician-in-Chief, A.I. DuPont Hospital for Children*

"The breakthrough book of a generation for brain change and a real blueprint of hope."

—*Cynthia Frisina, Founder, Reaching for the Stars, Atlanta, GA*

"Accessible insights into breakthroughs in the understanding of neurological deficits in children, and exciting additions to the repertoire of available treatment methods."

—*Warwick J. Peacock, MD, Director of the Surgical Science Laboratory at UCLA, Professor Emeritus Neurosurgery, UCSF*

"Never before has a book been written that so effectively marries science and story to help parents understand how they can improve their child's potential."

—*Professor Iona Novak, PhD, Head of Research, Research Institute,*
Cerebral Palsy Alliance, The University of Sydney, Australia

"Dr. Pape's recognition of this potential of the brain as it can be reflected in improved movement after brain damage, when the important authorities in medicine and neuroscience research strongly held the opposite belief, is a signal achievement and testament to her intellectual courage."

—*Professor Edward Taub, PhD, Director, CI Therapy Research Group*
and Taub Training Clinic, Birmingham, AL

"As an adult with cerebral palsy, I kept yelling, "YES! YES!" as I read *The Boy Who Could Run But Not Walk*. Finally, a book written by a doctor who 'gets it' when it comes to cerebral palsy treatment."

—*John W. Quinn, author of* Someone Like Me: An Unlikely Story of
Challenge and Triumph Over Cerebral Palsy

"An amazing book that proves habit hides recovery. It can be done; it doesn't matter what the disability. A good therapist, parent, or a sports coach can train a patient like an athlete—to achieve an optimal level of performance."

—*Karen Orlando, BSc, PT, Diploma Sport Physiotherapy, and member*
of the Canadian Olympic and Paralympic medical teams

"A brilliantly insightful, contemporary, must-read on the practical applications of basic neuroscience discoveries."

—*Elizabeth Theriault, PhD, Vice President Research and Informatics,*
Ontario Brain Institute

"This book has changed my expectations of what a child with brain injury can accomplish, and the results are truly astonishing."

—*Pia Stampe, PT, DPT, Step by Step Pediatric Therapy Center, Rochester, NY*

"A wonderful journey through Pape's career and scientific philosophy of neuroplasticity. Revelatory. Her greatest revelation may be that 'habits hide recovery'—poor motor strategies adopted by an injured nervous system

"Dr. Karen Pape challenges the 'can't do' attitudes surrounding traditional treatment. As parents, we can do no less."

—*Ron Dolenti and Hope Caldwell, parents of twin boys with cerebral palsy*

"Thank you, Dr. Karen Pape, for filling a void for parents who face the vast and intimidating landscape of therapies for children with cerebral palsy. *The Boy Who Could Run But Not Walk* will be my go-to guide for many years to come."

—*Shoshana Hahn-Goldberg, PhD, mother of child with cerebral palsy*

"When my son was 10, the medical field and therapists were unsure and lacking any hope for him to achieve new function or improve. He works out *every day*, played a whole season of sled hockey, and is more comfortable with his body than he has ever been! An absolute *must*-read for parents, physicians, and therapists!"

—*Ruth Grant-Bailey, BSN, RN, mother to Mason Bailey, age 16*

"Like Norman Doidge and Oliver Sacks, Karen Pape challenges medical orthodoxy and breaks new ground. Her work should be required reading for medical students, practicing physicians, physiotherapists, and anyone who works with, coaches, cares for, and loves someone with cerebral palsy."

—*Norah Myers, writer and editor*

"In my late-30s, I was told that I'd never walk unaided again. Dr. Karen Pape had the audacity to believe otherwise. My wish is that this book will encourage doctors not to settle for the status quo, but to look beyond the disabilities they see."

—*Catherine Bell, President, PRIME Impressions, and polio survivor*

"Dr. Karen Pape changes the paradigm 'No hope of a cure' to 'Cure for some and improvement for all,' giving children with brain damage a reason to fight."

—*Lorenzo Beltrame, professional tennis player and coach, awarded Coach of the Year and "Doc" Counsilman Science Awards by the United States Olympic Committee* may preclude further improvements possible in a more mature or recovered nervous system."

—*Keith Tansey, MD, PhD, Professor, Departments of Neurosurgery and Neurobiology, University of Mississippi Medical Center, and President-Elect, American Spinal Injury Association*

"Refreshing and energizing! *The Boy Who Could Run But Not Walk* leads us on a journey not only of hope, but of action."

—*Suzanne Davis Bombria, PT, C/NDT, Coordinator-Instructor, CT*

"Read this book. Dr. Karen Pape offers us the benefit of her remarkable and at times frustrating journey as a neonatologist who would not allow her own unorthodox understanding of the nervous system to be swallowed by conventional medical practices."

—*Harris A. Gelbard, MD, PhD, Director, Center for Neural Development and Disease, University of Rochester Medical Center, and Wendy B. Gelbard, MD, Associate Vice President Student Affairs, Rochester Institute of Technology*

"Finally, hope can be passed on to the masses of parents and individuals needing to train smarter and pursue great therapies with success. This book will change lives."

—*Ross Lilley, Executive Director/Founder, AccesSportAmerica, Boston, MA*

"A solid education in brain injury recovery for the layperson, reminding parents to re-think what they have been told about their child's prognosis."

—*Deb Discenza, Founder, CEO, Publisher, Preemie World, LLC*

"The potential for improvement, and even cure, for children with CP and other forms of brain injury appears to be grossly under exploited. *The Boy Who Could Run But Not Walk* offers genuine hope for all parents of at risk and diagnosed children with cerebral palsy."

—*Drew Smith, PhD, Director, Motion Analysis Research Center, Samuel Merritt University, Oakland, CA*

THE

BOY

WHO

COULD

RUN

BUT NOT WALK

Understanding Neuroplasticity in the Child's Brain

Karen Pape, MD

with Jonathan Webb

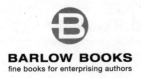

BARLOW BOOKS
fine books for enterprising authors

Library and Archives Canada Cataloguing in Publication data available upon
request.

ISBN 978-1-988025-05-6 (hardcover)
ISBN 978-1-988025-06-3 (ebook)

Printed in Canada

TO ORDER:
In Canada:
    Georgetown Publications
    34 Armstrong Avenue, Georgetown, ON L7G 4R9

In the U.S.A.:
    Midpoint Book Sales & Distribution
    27 West 20th Street, Suite 1102, New York, NY 10011

Cover design: Margie Miller
Cover illustration: Eladora, Shutterstock/123RF
Interior design and page layout: Kyle Gell Design

For more information, visit **www.barlowbooks.com**

BARLOW
BOOKS

Barlow Book Publishing Inc.
96 Elm Avenue, Toronto, ON
Canada M4W 1P2

*For my teachers and mentors, who taught me
to ask questions, and for the thousands of patients
and their families, who were my greatest resource
throughout my career.*

*With love to Sarah and Aaron, the best children
anyone could ever hope to have.*

contents

The information in this book is based on my years of clinical practice and research, and represents my best interpretation of the natural history of early acquired brain or nerve injuries. It is a comprehensive interpretation of my current knowledge, but I do not claim it to be complete. The information on medical conditions, therapy practices, and procedures is provided to the reader with the sole aim of developing your personal skills as an informed consumer. If you feel that any of my suggestions may apply to your child or yourself, please first discuss any action with your health-care team. Neither the author nor the publisher shall be liable or responsible for any loss or damage thought to arise from any information or suggestions in this book.

The clinical stories in this book are true. In some cases, names have been changed and stories have been merged to protect patient confidentiality. All direct quotes from patients or parents are included with their express permission to use both names and their story.

Products or procedures or surgeries mentioned in this book are for information only and should not be taken as a guarantee or endorsement.

At the date of publication, both the author and publisher have made every effort to ensure that information and internet addresses are accurate. Neither the author nor the publisher can be held responsible for changes to the contents or addresses of any external sites after publication.

Starting a Revolution

In the late 1990s, a three-year-old girl had half her brain surgically removed. She had Rasmussen's syndrome, an inflammation of the brain that causes seizures that get progressively worse. Her seizures were not responding to medication and the damage was affecting her language skills and motor control. She was losing the ability to speak and the right side of her body was tightening up. Her condition was bad and getting worse.

By taking out the affected half of her brain, the surgeons expected to stop the seizures. They assumed she would remain disabled. They thought she might or might not be able to speak, but they were pretty sure she would achieve a degree of mobility. She would likely require a brace on one ankle (on the side opposite the half of her brain that was removed) to help her walk. But she would be alive and managing, and that, in the circumstances, was something.

What they did not anticipate is what actually happened.

The little girl recovered completely.

Not only were her seizures eradicated, but by the time she was seven she was running about like any other child. Her arm and hand were a bit stiff, but not enough to be noticeable. And, to top it off, even though the speech centres in her left brain had been removed, she was bilingual, fluent in Turkish and Dutch. All the functions that she should have lost, according to orthodox theory, had been restored.

She was just fine.[1]

———— • ————

There are other isolated cases in the medical literature that are no less remarkable.

Over thirty-five years ago, a physician in Sheffield, England, noticed that one of his students had a larger than usual head. It wasn't grotesque, but it was something a doctor would notice and this doctor was curious. He referred the young man to John Lorber, a professor of pediatrics at Sheffield University. Lorber ran a brain scan on the young man and what he saw was astounding. The average thickness of an adult human brain is approximately four and a half centimetres on each side between the outer cortical surface and the fluid-filled ventricles in the centre. In this young man with an enlarged head, the ventricles were huge and the brain tissue, the part that allows us to think and move, had been compressed to a tiny one-millimetre sliver of brain tissue.[2]

The young man's problem was caused by hydrocephalus, a condition in which excess fluid builds up in the head. In this case, the blockage causing the fluid build-up was incomplete, so the pressure in the young man's head increased slowly over time from a young age. In children, the skull bones separate and grow larger in response to the build-up of fluid, producing the large-looking head first noticed by his doctor. The brain tissue was able to compensate by stretching and thinning out. He probably still had a "normal" amount of brain tissue, but its shape and distribution had changed.

One might think that stretching and thinning a brain would affect the mental functioning of the young man. But no. He was thought to have an IQ of 126, had achieved first-class honours in mathematics, and was by all accounts leading an entirely conventional everyday life.

————— • —————

These two outstanding examples show that even if a person loses half a brain, and even when the brain is compressed to a one-millimetre sliver, it can still function, and function pretty well. One patient had a higher than normal IQ; the other spoke two very different languages. The young brain can change. This is neuroplasticity.

These cases were not, to say the least, what doctors expected. Until recently, the prevailing theory has been that the brain cannot change. If some part of it is injured, the part of the body it controls will also be damaged forever. Yet doctors will quietly admit that they do see cases that contradict the traditional theory about the brain. These cases might not be as dramatic as the girl who learned to speak Turkish and Dutch with only half a brain, but they show that even after a brain injury, a child can sometimes do things that no one expects. So how does the medical establishment deal with the cases that don't fit the official story?

Largely, they are ignored. If physicians do pay attention to them, these extraordinary stories are dismissed as outliers. They don't count.

It turns out that most physicians and scientists have difficulty with cases that don't fit in with mainstream thinking. Even when the anomalies are brought to their attention by an unimpeachable source, they tend to shrug philosophically and confess that, you know, sometimes things happen that we can't explain. Or they might think they don't have the full story: data might be missing, the experimental model could be faulty, or the facts could have been misinterpreted. More often, they simply ignore the outliers and carry on working within the system as it stands, assuring anyone who asks that it has served them just fine, thank you very much, and they're not about to change it. This happens all the time.

Why?

Thomas Kuhn, an American physicist and philosopher of science, explains why outliers, in all fields of scientific endeavour, are often ignored. In *The Structure of Scientific Revolutions*, first published in 1962,[3] he explains that normal science, that is, the day-to-day work of scientific research done by most scientists, most of the time, rests on the acceptance of a broad understanding of the way things work. Outliers are ignored until researchers stumble upon so many inconvenient observations that they can't ignore them anymore. For as long as they possibly can, they carry on with science as it's come to be understood.

Picture a scattergram with a straight line drawn through it. The line represents the explanatory theory; the dots represent data. When the theory is new, almost all the dots are clustered close to the line: the theory is doing a satisfactory job of explaining the data. The distance between the line and the dots indicates the standard deviation from the mean: it's expected. Physicists exploring water turbulence, meteorologists attempting to predict the weather, and so on, all know that there is variation. Not all data fit the theory perfectly. But as long as most of the data support the theory, the outliers can be discounted.

That is, until so many data points veer away from the mean that they can't be ignored and the accepted theory becomes insupportable.

— • —

Kuhn's insights apply to what I was taught about brain injury in humans in medical school and later in pediatric training. For a very long time, doctors and neuroscientists thought that human brain damage was permanent and irreversible. The occasional outliers like the little girl with half a brain were dismissed as fortunate exceptions to the rule that human brains had limited ability to change and heal. In the latter part of the twentieth century, the medical world discovered and gradually accepted a revolutionary new idea: our brains can regrow new cells, repair injuries, rewire new connections, and reallocate brain resources to restore lost function. This was neuroplasticity, and it sparked a true scientific revolution. It has shaken up many areas of medicine, especially adult neurology. As a result of improvements in diagnosis, early treatment, and later rehabilitation for adults with stroke, up to 30 percent of people with a first-time, mild stroke now may have a complete recovery, and *their outlook is improving all the time*.

Yet a baby with a similar stroke, with a brain injury in the same area of the brain as the adult, is expected to have the abnormal movement patterns that we associate with cerebral palsy (CP) for life. The official position of the National Institutes of Health in the United States that provides the most up-to-date information on neurologic diseases still maintains that cerebral palsy is a *permanent* disorder of movement and a condition with *no* cure.[4]

It makes no sense: an adult with a mild stroke may recover completely, but a baby with a similar mild stroke will not recover and instead have a permanent disorder of movement and posture called cerebral palsy. Changing the name of a condition from stroke to cerebral palsy does not change the reality that a young, growing brain should have a better chance of full recovery than an old, deteriorating brain.

I have spent my career as a neonatologist and clinical neuroscientist trying to understand this apparent contradiction.

After training in pediatrics, I specialized in neonatology, caring for premature babies born early and full-term infants with complications arising from problems at or near the time of birth. During their stay in the Neonatal Intensive Care Unit (NICU), some of these babies developed various types of brain injury, documented on brain scans. I encountered a small number of outliers, babies with clear-cut damage to their brains who unexpectedly recovered completely. Those babies who recovered were and still are considered anomalies by most of my colleagues, but I saw so many of them that I became convinced the anomalies were actually the story, just as Kuhn had suggested.

These outliers prove, beyond any reasonable doubt, that baby brains can change and heal, even more than adult brains can. It explains why the boy with cerebral palsy whom I once treated can run but not walk properly. When he learned to walk, his brain was still damaged, so he developed an awkward walking gait. Yet by the time he learned to run, the parts of his brain that controlled both walking and running had healed and matured. So he could run like the other boys could. He could run, but his walking was still hampered, not by brain damage but by bad habits, just like the bad habits that plague the 22-handicap golfer.

It is time to reassess how neuroplasticity is expressed in the baby and young child. That is what this book is about: the anomalies that do not fit the prevailing theory that baby brain injuries are permanent and irreversible. Improving the outcome for these children will have a huge impact on childhood disability. Most people do not know that cerebral palsy is the most common motor disorder of childhood. There are close to a million cases of CP in the United States, with 17 million or more worldwide. This number translates into approximately one new diagnosis of CP made every hour in the United States.

This book is the story of how my colleagues and I gradually put together a new explanation of how early brain injury leads to the motor impairments that are collectively called cerebral palsy. Working with young children with documented brain injuries at or shortly after birth, I kept noticing the outliers, the children who functioned more or less normally despite having badly altered brains. Yet a question that took years to answer was why the motor problems of children diagnosed later with CP were so persistent. How could we fix long-established bad habits?

Throughout my career, I have been fortunate to have been taught by gifted teachers, mentors, and also parents of children with cerebral palsy who insisted their child was doing better than their doctors (including me) thought was possible. We found that we needed a different approach to both diagnosis and therapy for children with CP and other forms of early brain damage.

Many of the proven breakthrough treatments and adjustments to the existing system for treating children and adults with cerebral palsy draw on what we have learned from adult neurologic research and exercise science. We have found that this new approach has positive implications, not only for children and adults with the wide range of problems that are included within a cerebral palsy diagnosis, but also for patients with spinal cord injury, brachial plexus injury, and even post-polio syndrome. We know now that even severely affected children can expect some improvement. For those whose disability is mild, there is real hope of a full recovery. I have seen it happen. In these pages, you will too.

one

The Boy Who Could Run But Not Walk

first saw Daniel as a premature infant when I was a neo-natology fellow at the Hospital for Sick Children (HSC, or Sick Kids) in Toronto. Daniel was born at twenty-six weeks. In the first week of his life, he developed a major bleed into the right side of his brain, damaging the areas that would normally control the left side of his body.

A twenty-six-week infant is tiny. Daniel at birth weighed 750 grams, about a pound and a half. When I started in neonatology in the 1970s, he would have had, at best, about a fifty-fifty chance of surviving. Daniel survived, but the common wisdom at the time was that the damage to his brain was permanent and would lead to disability. The expectation was that he would have difficulty with both gross and fine motor skills. We knew he had a brain lesion so he was started in therapy fairly early. To my surprise, the disabilities that developed in Daniel as he grew from infancy to childhood, as measured on a standardized scale of function, were not too bad. As I expected, he limped on the left side, landing on the front half of his foot, not his heel. His left arm hung at his side and did not swing normally when he walked. His right side was unaffected and his speech and cognition were normal. I diagnosed him with a left-sided hemiplegia, a type of cerebral palsy that affects the motor functions just on one side of the body. Hemiplegia is found in roughly 40 percent of all children with cerebral palsy, and, like Daniel, 99 percent of these children are able to walk.[1]

The Neonatal Follow-Up Clinic, where I worked, tracked patients for only the first three to four years. Daniel had been discharged for several years when his mother phoned me with news. She told me he was now playing soccer, not just in a league that accepted children of diverse ability, but in a league for competitive, able-bodied children.

The hell he is, I thought.

What I said was, "Oh?"

I didn't believe her. Daniel being able to play competitive soccer was outside my understanding of hemiplegia. I assumed, as many doctors would have, that an overly optimistic mother was seeing a degree of recovery that just wasn't there. Still, I arranged for her to come in with Daniel so I could see for myself. When they came, I had him walk up and down the hallway to confirm that he still had the typical gait of a child with mild spastic hemiplegia. He did.

Then I asked him to run.

And, to my astonishment, he ran like a normal little boy, with an easy, balanced stride and reciprocal arm movements. He performed tight pivot turns, at speed, on both legs. Even the left leg, which had a limp when he walked, performed perfectly when he was running.

For a moment I was speechless. (Anyone who knows me knows this rarely happens.) Then I said, "You can't do that!" And I meant it. I could not, for the life of me, figure out what was going on. We all know children learn to walk before they run. It's a phrase embedded in folk wisdom. And yet, here was a child who had turned conventional wisdom upside down.

My first instinct was to think of Daniel as an outlier, an exception who somehow defied the rules. The natural history of cerebral palsy has been studied and described over a period of decades, and Daniel's ability to run so well didn't fit the description. It was incomprehensible in terms of the accepted theory of permanent brain damage that my fellow physicians and I understood. Which is why I said, "You can't do that!" What he was doing was impossible.

—— • ——

Daniel's ability to run was great for him but it posed a problem for me and, indeed, for anyone treating children with cerebral palsy. We walk and run using the same parts of our brain. Daniel's brain—specifically the corticospinal system on the left side of his brain that controls movement—was injured, so I thought there was no way he could run.

But he could run really well.

(He could also turn at speed and kick a soccer ball accurately with either leg, but, frankly, his running was enough of an issue without my having to take these added abilities into account.)

It took many years for me to realize that our assumptions of permanent brain damage were wrong and his normal run meant that his brain had recovered from the early injury. The damage had been repaired. Or the brain had grown and its capacity had grown with it. Or new neural pathways had been forged in his brain to get around the original damage. In the late 1970s, these were all new ideas when it came to thinking about the outcome of brain injury in newborns. The idea that the brain can grow, adapt, and recover from damage has been the subject of research and debate for many years, but the majority of research into neuroplasticity had been in animal studies or adult human diseases and injuries.[2] As far as I knew, very few people had speculated that an infant's brain could heal itself as the child grew up. It didn't occur to me then either. All I had when I saw Daniel run were questions.

What is going on?

How is this possible?

—— • ——

Once I had noticed the discrepancy between Daniel's poor walking skills and his superior running skills, I started to see more examples. Most experienced therapists can help a child with mild cerebral palsy produce, in as little as a one-hour session, a short-distance walk with a perfectly acceptable, heel-to-toe reciprocal gait. In North America, this is frequently called a "therapy walk." To the endless frustration of both therapists and parents, the child who has laboriously acquired a new way of walking in the therapy session loses it on the way to the parking lot for the trip home. The more familiar unsteady gait of the child with hemiplegia reasserts itself.

Even the children know the difference between their therapy walk and their habitual walk. When asked to demonstrate their "best walk," most children with mild cerebral palsy will straighten up and walk normally. They have been drilled by their therapists and have practised these correct movements many times. When asked to demonstrate their regular walk, they happily go back to the abnormal gait that is their comfortable habit. If you ask why they do not keep walking as they have been taught, they say it doesn't feel normal to them. They can do it, but it doesn't feel comfortable. For Daniel, his limping gait was his normal. What the therapist taught him felt weird.

Over years of clinical practice, I have found that most children with mild to moderate cerebral palsy run better than they walk. This fact is known by most experienced therapists, orthopedic surgeons, and physicians, but they, like me, did not stop to think it through. If the run is normal, if the therapy walk is ever normal, even briefly, then the corticospinal system must have recovered.

Thirty-five years after treating Daniel, it is now obvious to me that children with early neurologic damage can have two or more completely different skill levels all originating from the same area of the brain. There are thousands of children just like him. A mother sent me a soccer card of her son, the kind of imitation bubble-gum card that professional photographers make when they take pictures of children in organized sports. It showed that her boy, diagnosed with the same kind of CP as Daniel, was playing soccer too. I saw children with cerebral palsy who rode bicycles, who skateboarded and ice-skated. Even roller-blading, a skill I would not even attempt, was not beyond the reach of a young boy from California who did not let the diagnosis of spastic cerebral palsy hold him back. This young boy could walk only with an unsteady, lurching gait that is characteristic of diplegia, affecting the motor control of both legs, yet he was able to roller-blade with skill. I met another boy with hemiplegia who was playing on his high school basketball team. He could run, turn, jump, and pivot and even throw the ball accurately using both hands. I learned later that he went on to coach the sport.

Probably the biggest shock was a teenager with mild athetoid quadriplegia (meaning all four limbs were involved, with significant coordination and balance problems) who won a gold medal at a swim meet in the butterfly event. For those who are not swimmers, this is a stroke that defeats many an able-bodied swimmer. Her parents showed me videos of her competing. She would walk up to the starting block with all the awkwardness associated with her condition and then swim like a dolphin. In a variety of ways, children with CP were showing me that their hemiplegia, diplegia, and even mild quadriplegia, obvious when they walked, disappeared when they took part in challenging higher-order activities.

I got another surprise when the mother of a little girl made an unexpected observation. We were watching her daughter walk in the hall of the clinic. By this time I had made walking and running in the hallway a routine part of my initial examination of every patient who was able to walk. She had spastic hemiplegia: she could bring the affected leg only about half as far forward as the unaffected leg. The medical term for this is a shortened stride length.

"She walks better backwards," said her mother.

What? It's not something you think of ordinarily. How often do we walk backwards?

I said, "Show me." The child backed up as easily as an able-bodied person would, with no sign of spasticity, perfectly balanced. She had a normal stride length on both sides.

We walk and run with the same parts of the brain. This means that the highest-order or "best" skill reflects the degree to which the brain has recovered from the early injury. The lower skill level is the habit acquired when the brain was still damaged. When I saw Daniel run, what I was seeing was definite evidence of brain recovery. And when I saw him walk, I was witnessing a well-established habit that is not easily shed.

I now understand that many of the early-learned movements of a child with cerebral palsy are habits. And habits can only be replaced with new ones with difficulty. But they can be replaced.

— • —

I had some experience with habits in my own life. I started playing tennis with my grandfather the summer I was four years old. I could barely hit a ball sent directly at me, but I tried and was happy with anything that worked. I wasn't worried about the best way to hit the ball; I was just trying to get it over the net. Not surprisingly, right from the start, my forehand technique was terrible, and it stayed that way. I had a habit of hitting the ball into the net. When I was tired or stressed, it got even worse.

Years later, my coach came up with a remedy. He strung a cord eighteen inches above the net, setting a new goal for me by changing the rules of the game. Instead of hitting the ball on a downward trajectory, which had become my habit, I had to send it higher, using a different combination of muscles in an altered sequence of moves. When, after I had practised this new skill for days on end, he took the cord down, my forehand was stronger and faster and the ball consistently cleared the net. He had given me an altered and, in tennis terms, improved way of moving. And that was all he cared about. But in order to do this, he had made me forge new wired-in neural circuits that determined how my hand, arm, shoulder, torso—in fact, how my entire body—responded in a quick, instinctive manner to the approaching tennis ball. Because hitting a tennis ball, like any other physical movement, is not just a matter involving muscles, tendons, and bones: it also engages the sensory and motor control centres in the brain. It's a complex, reciprocal circuit, all of it firing much faster than thought. My coach didn't just change my tennis stroke. He changed my brain.

There are parallels between a practised motor movement in an athlete or a musician and a child with cerebral palsy. Athletes and coaches call a practised movement "muscle memory." Neuroscientists call it a "facilitated brain network." It is an easy jump to think about Daniel's walk and run in these terms. His habitual hemiplegic walk feels normal to him, whereas walking as most people do feels wrong. Any athlete knows this feeling. It comes on whenever she tries to change a maladaptive pattern of movement that was learned early into something more advanced and functional in her sport. Focused, purposeful practice of the new motor pattern is needed to change what feels like an awkward movement into a new brain-body habit.

When I first encountered Daniel, changing habits was not one of my skill sets. We weren't given much guidance in medical school about how to help people change. As a profession, doctors often urge their patients to quit smoking, lose weight, and reduce their alcohol consumption for the sake of their health. But our advice is rarely combined with an effective program. And people find it really hard to quit smoking, stick to a diet, or reduce their alcohol intake. Coaches, however, are engaged in either establishing good habits or curing their athletes of bad ones all the time. It's what they do. And what they do, however unintentionally, is exploit the principles of neuroplasticity. They're unlikely to use the term, and they rarely if ever explain what they're doing in language a neuroscientist would employ. But, regardless, they understand how to train both the body and the brain. Winning depends on it. And their job is to win.

My coach gave my brain a challenge when he raised the height of the net by eighteen inches. If you want to fully engage the power of the brain to alter behaviour, you have to give it something new to do. Neuroplasticity is stimulated by novel, challenging tasks. Without novelty and challenge, well-established habits always dominate. If the new task assigned to the brain is repeated often enough, then the behaviour becomes instinctive and almost effortless. The neurons fire along new pathways. As the paths are pounded down by neural traffic, they get wider, smoother, and easier to follow. Metaphorically, the paths become roads and the roads become highways. Technically (sort of) they are paved with white matter—a substance called myelin—that reinforces neural highways, increasing the speed of transmission. These highways become the brain's default route when a particular action is performed. This default pathway is facilitated by use. The term "facilitated" means that frequently fired neural networks (habits) become easier to activate. This is the underlying neuroscience insight that explains how habits are formed.

— • —

Daniel experienced his brain hemorrhage in the first weeks of his life. How long does it take for the baby brain to recover from a birth trauma? We don't know. No one has figured out how to answer this important question. We do know, however, that adults with a stroke may continue to show improvement and restoration of function for three to four years. Assuming the same pattern applies to children, Daniel learned to walk in the first few years when his brain was in the process of recovery from the early bleed into the primary motor control part of the brain called the corticospinal system. In these early years, when the child has a relatively immature brain, he can access only the damaged corticospinal system to learn how to sit, crawl, and walk. It was in this period that Daniel's left-sided spasticity developed and he adopted the typical gait of a child with hemiplegia.

Gradually, however, Daniel's brain recovered. It grew and matured. Between three and six years, there's a significant development in all children: the cerebellum comes online. The cerebellum can be thought of as a backup system for the rest of the brain. It coordinates and refines motor movements, particularly rapid, alternating movements. The child with mild to moderate cerebral palsy, who up to this point has been somewhat clumsy with poor balance, can now learn to run, jump, and climb with a very different brain from the one that he was using in the first two to three years. The brain has had time to recover and it is now considerably more sophisticated.

Children learn all the basic gross motor skills in the early period. Any improvement after four years is due to skill training. Daniel was up and running by four years, as are almost all children with mild hemiplegia. It was when he was six that he started to play soccer. For the six-year-old child with a more mature and recovered brain, the maladaptive, awkward walk is a kind of vestige: it's a habit formed with a damaged, immature brain. And like any habit, it's hard to get rid of. The later-learned, higher-order skills, honed on the soccer field, are the ones that show the extent of brain recovery. The old saying that you have to learn to walk before you can run does not apply to the child with an early neurologic problem. On the contrary, before he can run well, he has to wait for his brain to catch up.

—— • ——

The observation that much of the maladaptive movement patterns associated with cerebral palsy can be looked at as habits came to me slowly. One of the clues came from my tennis coach, who gave me a new way to think about my forehand. He showed me that a bad habit can be changed. My new understanding also came from the exciting findings in the emerging field of practical brain science.

In the 1980s, University of California neuroscientist Michael Merzenich challenged the long-established view that each activity was directed by a specific part of the brain. If that were true, brain damage to a specific part of the brain would cause irreversible damage. The implications of the traditional line of thinking for CP were profound. It suggested that when a baby brain was damaged, it was damaged for life. Children would never be able to walk normally.

However, Merzenich was one of the earliest scientists to flat out disprove that theory. In a series of experiments, Merzenich and his colleagues damaged the sensory nerves connecting a monkey's hand to the brain. They wanted to study what would happen to the parts of the brain normally activated by the now absent sensory nerves. What he saw was extraordinary: the surrounding parts of the brain moved into the unused section of the brain lacking its sensory nerve. This study proved that each part of the brain did not, as scientists previously thought, have a permanent assignment. The brain could and did change. The brain is efficiency driven and will co-opt unused brain real estate and put it to work on other tasks.

It was a clear demonstration that the brain can reorganize function in response to trauma.

To me, the even more exciting finding was that as the trauma to the sensory nerve resolved, the brain reorganized back to its original form and functioned once again. Merzenich demonstrated conclusively that the adult animal brain could rewire or change itself. What's more, the way it rewires is determined by the input it receives. When the input from the monkey's hand to the brain declined, the sensory part of the brain became smaller. When the nerve recovered and sensory input was restored, the brain returned to its pre-injury size. Merzenich called this "activity-dependent neuroplasticity." It's a mechanism that explains a lot and one that—as Merzenich himself has demonstrated—can be put to practical use.[3] His research has been wide-ranging, from the early work of developing cochlear implants to give hearing to babies born deaf, to brain training to cancel out certain types of learning disability and proven exercises to retrain and restore the aging human brain. His work in the latter part of the twentieth century demonstrated that brains can change. The old concept of a fixed, computer-like brain was wrong.

— • —

For the longest time, I didn't see the signs that the brain had recovered. I didn't see the children run because, knowing how they walked, I didn't think to ask if they could run. Realistically, most offices and clinics don't have much room for running. I didn't see them walk backwards because with the obvious difficulty they experienced walking forwards, why would I ask them to walk backwards? Their abnormal, maladaptive walk, a habit acquired when their brain was injured, was my focus. Their ability to develop stronger, better balanced behaviour patterns with their recovered, more mature brain was basically ignored as an unexplained phenomenon. The maladaptive behaviour concealed it from us.

Habit hides recovery.

I eventually concluded that, when it comes to children with early brain injury, we have to assess them in a different way. Doctors and therapists are trained to look at the walk, see what is wrong about a movement, and then try to fix it. It took me a long time to train myself to seek out what the child *could do*. This is the child's highest skill level, the level that reveals the level of brain recovery.

Once you know there is a maladaptive habit interfering with a child's ability to achieve a higher skill level in a particular task, you have to be inventive. Habits are not broken or changed; they are replaced. Trying to gradually change a maladaptive walking habit while a therapist gives instructions from the sidelines to "lift your knees" or "keep your heels down" actually activates and strengthens the abnormal movement circuit. At first this sounds counterintuitive. I thought focusing the child's attention on what was wrong with the walk would help him learn a new way of walking. However, all it does is reinforce the old habit.

What's happening inside the brain that is trying to change an old habit? It's almost impossible for a scan to show how the brain controls the process of walking or running, since the patient must stay still to take the scan. However, a brain scan can show what happens when the patient *thinks* about moving. Individuals who have obsessive-compulsive disorder (OCD) often develop repetitive patterns of movement that help reduce their anxiety. Repeated thousands and thousands of times, this movement pattern becomes a facilitated network in their brains. It has been demonstrated by functional brain scans in adult patients with OCD that their brains light up in specific areas when they just think about doing a habitual routine. The surprising finding was that their brains light up even more when they think of *not* performing the behaviour. The effort of trying to inhibit a facilitated network actually fires the network and makes it stronger!

It took me a long time to understand that impairments that develop after an initial brain injury were habits that might be prevented, and that bad habits can be replaced by new, more functional habits. This was a new way of seeing children with early neurologic injury. I began to think this way largely because the way I was trained and educated was very different from the way most physicians are trained. Looking back now, I realize how lucky I was to have had world-class teachers and mentors who each contributed to my understanding of how neuroplasticity rewires the young brain. Their stories follow next.

two

The Heretical Teachers

I was taught early in my career that our brains have a remarkable ability to recover function after an injury. Psychologists and psychiatrists had long recognized this fact, but sadly, in medical fields the prevailing doctrine was that human brains had limited potential. Simply stated, we were born with all the nerve cells we would have for life. If damaged, there was no possibility of recovery. Human neuroplasticity is now an accepted scientific fact, and its acceptance has transformed adult brain, spinal cord, and nerve injury rehabilitation.

Unfortunately, the pediatric world has still not fully accepted the neuroplasticity revolution. A perfect example comes from one of the most trusted sources for up-to-date information about brains, the National Institute of Neurological Disorders and Stroke, or NINDS for short. This eminent institution publishes web pages that provide current information about all the different diseases and disorders of the brain. On the cerebral palsy page, NINDS offers this depressing outlook for children with brain damage that results in cerebral palsy: *"Cerebral palsy can't be cured*, but treatment will often improve a child's capabilities."[1] Yet the outlook is far better for adults who have brain damage that produces the characteristic abnormal movement pattern of a stroke: "New advances in imaging and rehabilitation have shown that *the brain can compensate for function lost as a result of stroke.*"[2]

It is a study in contrasting worldviews.

The stroke page contains up-to-date information that recognizes the reality of human neuroplasticity. Unfortunately, in 2016, the cerebral palsy page still conforms to an outdated, pre-neuroplasticity dogma. It is time for pediatric neurorehabilitation, the specialty area that primarily cares for children with early brain damage, to move into the twenty-first century.

Pediatric neurorehabilitation is a comparatively young specialty. There were no formal training positions when I started out, and as a result, most of us learned our skills "on the job," drawn to the care of children with cerebral palsy for many different reasons. Unfortunately, most of what we learned about treatment and the prognosis for change was developed over the last half of the twentieth century in the pre-neuroplasticity era. These outdated beliefs no longer accurately reflect what is now known about early neurologic injury and the potential for recovery in children.

It is time to challenge our underlying assumptions about the possibility of recovery and develop new ways of thinking about prognosis. I want to give children themselves and the people who care for them hope. Not hope for a miracle or an amazing breakthrough sometime in the far-off future. What I have in mind is hope that we can change what we do right now, using the knowledge and tools that are available. This is *real hope*.

Unfortunately, scientific revolutions are disruptive and are actively resisted by the guardians of the past. As a result, I have spent a lot of time arguing with the status quo. I have often been described as a "difficult" person. The people I most admire have often been difficult too. You have to be a bit difficult to start a revolution, to make things happen. I was fortunate to have as mentors and friends a succession of men and women who were willing, when the occasion demanded it, to be difficult.

— • —

The path charted for me by these pioneers was a winding and unconventional one. My first medical mentor was Walter Hannah, a young obstetrician at Women's College Hospital in Toronto. For two summers, in 1960 and 1961, I lied about my age and got a job as a clerk in the Outpatient Department, filling in for a pair of elderly ladies who each took a long vacation. The work was boring and I was able to get through it in an hour or two, so I asked permission to read patients' medical charts. This led me to ask questions—What does this mean? Why was that done?—and the head nurse got tired of answering them. She introduced me to Dr. Hannah, who was doing a research study that meant he had to review the day's obstetrics charts each afternoon. He agreed to indulge my curiosity. Not many physicians would have been so generous, but Hannah was a remarkable man. By my second summer as the clinic clerk, he was letting me observe medical procedures.

My continued chart-reading taught me that the charts often described a flawed process: each entry was perfectly sensible, based on the data that were immediately available, but real problems became apparent when you read the chart through from beginning to end. There were false trails pursued and then abandoned, as well as misdiagnoses and errors in medication. Hannah was tickled when I pointed them out and he set about correcting them.

Most physicians don't have time to review a history as thoroughly as I did when I read those charts. But to me, they were like a mystery novel (which I also enjoy reading). They gave me the chance to see what was happening over time. I was fascinated by what I learned and I became hooked on both the science and practice of medicine. This early introduction to medical records and research had a long-lasting impact on me. Years later, when I was learning how to take a medical history, I always asked the patient to start at the beginning and tell me what had happened first. When was she last completely well? I had learned, reading charts from front to back, how important it was to know the whole history of the problem. It was the first step leading to my future career.

— • —

High schools in Ontario at that time required attendance over five years, grades nine through thirteen (this has since changed), while Quebec required only four. I seized on the discrepancy and applied to McGill University in Montreal from grade twelve. At McGill, I stumbled into a hotbed of new thinking about mind and brain function presided over by Donald Hebb. He taught the introductory psychology course, which was a course requirement for all first-year science students. He was the first to teach me that human brains can recover in adult life, even from devastating injuries. In a groundbreaking book, *The Organization of Behaviour*, published in 1949, Hebb described the history of a sixteen-year-old boy whose prefrontal lobes were removed by one of the pioneers of brain research, Wilder Penfield. The prefrontal lobes are thought to be the seat of abstract thought, planning, and decision making. You might think it would be hard to get by without them and, generally speaking, you would be right. They were removed to cure the young man of seizures and violent episodes that verged on psychotic. As it turned out, the cure was complete. According to Hebb, the young man, after the operation, was clinically and socially normal.[3]

Hebb's book wasn't chiefly about exceptional cases, however. It was about how the brain, with its billions of neurons and synapses, processes our thoughts, sensations, and emotions, as well as our physical actions. One of his most widely recognized theories concerns how brains change in response to activity. Hebb proposed that when an action is repeated, brain cells (neurons) fire in a way that is self-reinforcing, a process he called "cell assembly." Repetition of an action over time makes it happen faster and more readily. Hebb's description was dauntingly technical. "Let us assume then," he wrote, "that the persistence or repetition of a reverberatory activity (or 'trace') tends to induce lasting cellular changes that add to its stability. The assumption can be precisely stated as follows: *When an axon of cell A is near enough to excite a cell B and repeatedly or persistently takes part in firing it, some growth process or metabolic change takes place in one or both cells such that A's efficiency, as one of the cells firing B, is increased."*[4]

His description is technical but the idea at the heart of it is simple. Later commentators summed up the concept more succinctly than Hebb did himself. The phrase now associated with his theory is this: *neurons that fire together wire together*. This simple phrase has major implications. It means, for one thing, that brain processes that are often repeated eventually become hard-wired. They become more efficient, facilitated networks, or brain habits. For another, it implies that the brain can change if new neural networks are fired repetitively. This was a heretical concept at a time when most people used the metaphor of a hard-wired computer program to explain how brains work. Hebb's concept of *neurons that fire together wire together* stayed with me, although I did not understand its relationship to the boy who ran better than he walked for many years.

Hebb was a pioneer in his approach to understanding the workings of the brain and is considered by many to be the father of both neuropsychology and neural networks. He was a gifted teacher who encouraged us to challenge accepted dogma by example. By the time I left McGill, I knew with certainty that adult human brains could recover completely from devastating injury or surgeries and that they could change with use to become more efficient. Anything you do, your brain learns to do faster, using less energy.

I would soon find out what an outlier Hebb was. When I went to medical school, I was taught that human brains had limited neuroplasticity and what there was of it was only occasionally seen in the first years of life. Brain injury, according to the experts at medical school, was permanent and irreversible. Therapy after a brain injury consisted of teaching the person to compensate for lost function, not to restore it to the pre-injury level of function. Listening to all this, I still believed Hebb's theory that brains could change and recover, but I learned to keep my mouth shut.

—— • ——

In the McGill psychology department, Ronald Melzack, a protégé of Hebb, had a lasting impact on me but for a very different reason. Like Hebb, Melzack was interested in exploring the connections that linked mind and body. While I was still at McGill, Melzack and his long-time collaborator at the Massachusetts Institute of Technology, Patrick Wall, were working on their groundbreaking "gate" theory of pain, first published in *Science* in 1965.[5]

In the article, Melzack and Wall argued that pain happened in the brain rather than where it seemed to hurt. This helped to explain why an amputee felt pain in a limb that had been surgically removed. It was new, daring, and exciting stuff in the 1960s, and in Melzack's seminars, we read and discussed drafts of the article and chapters of their subsequent book, *The Textbook of Pain*, now in its sixth edition.[6]

Melzack was an inspired teacher and mentor. He introduced me to a new way of thinking about the way the body and the brain communicate, a frame of reference that would later help me to develop a new way of looking at cerebral palsy. He also talked to us about the resistance they were meeting as they tried to introduce this new approach into the established field of pain study. He taught me that not all new ideas are welcomed. Some are seen as a threat. It was an exciting peek into later battles to come, and I was blessed with a terrific teacher to show me the way.

In addition, he taught me a great deal more about pain than I learned later in medical school. In those days, pain was not a popular subject, and truthfully, we had few tools available to treat it. Years later, when I was a staff neonatologist at the Hospital for Sick Children, I was part of an initial morphine study in premature infants.[7] At that time, twenty years after my time at McGill, no pain relief was administered to babies during painful procedures. Before we could do the study, we had to get permission from the hospital ethics committee, and what we got was resistance. "Babies do not feel pain" was the dominant theory of care. I pointed out the harsh reality that when I put a needle into infants, they would hold their breath, screw up their face, and then cry out. "Looks and sounds like pain to me," I told them. We eventually got permission to do the study, but not until I had been told to "stop talking like a nurse." It was a clear instance of blind adherence to an outdated and incorrect theory. The nurses knew the babies were in pain. The doctors believed what they were taught and discounted the physiological changes that clearly indicated that the baby felt the pain. Even now, another thirty years later, babies' pain is still not widely treated, even in funded research trials reviewed by similar ethics committees.[8]

Another of my mentors at McGill, Dalbir Bindra, challenged B.F. Skinner's theory of operant conditioning. Skinner believed that behaviour was driven by a fairly direct reaction to repeated biological stimulus. A dog, for instance, will run in response to a whistle if the action is rewarded. Bindra, however, argued that our actions are more complex than Skinner's stimulus-response theory suggested. This seems terribly obvious now, but it was radical in the mid-1960s. His teachings were another example of a heretic marshalling evidence that went against the established theories of the period. He encouraged us to read widely and ask questions, to push the boundaries of what was known.

During my four years at McGill, I majored in experimental psychology and neurophysiology. In every course, the experimental design of each study was carefully scrutinized. Often, we were shown that the design was an inappropriate choice to answer the research question under study. I would not realize the importance of this part of my early training until later in my career.

— • —

Each summer while I attended McGill, I worked as a research assistant on different projects at Toronto's Clarke Institute of

Psychiatry (now the Centre for Addiction and Mental Health). The first year—to the distress of my family—I worked for the forensic psychology department, where, in addition to making notes from charts, I interviewed and performed various psychology tests as part of the legal remand process. I also took part in field trips to test a terrifying cross-section of mostly violent and disturbed criminals in a hospital for the criminally insane. This was useful experience in analyzing this sort of data and a sobering introduction to the dark side of the human personality.

The next year and the year after that, I was a junior research assistant for Bruce Quarrington, who was studying the nature of and treatments for speech impediments. His research showed that the problem was, to some degree, neurologic, but it could be affected by elements in the environment, such as the presence of strangers, and by personal factors, such as stress. With Dr. Quarrington, I learned that people who could speak normally when rested and in familiar surroundings could be reduced to painful speechlessness in front of strangers. It was obvious that if they could *ever* speak normally, the speech centres in their brain must be normal. The cause of their speech problem was to be found somewhere else and, in all likelihood, could be treated. The movie *The King's Speech* made much of this information more accessible to the general public, but I was surprised in my later training as a doctor that although I was taught how to diagnose different types of speech impairment, I was taught virtually nothing about treatment. My time with Dr. Quarrington was invaluable to my understanding of speech impairments in children with cerebral palsy.

Speech problems are found in roughly 25 percent of children with cerebral palsy, with a higher incidence in those with the more severe forms of the disorder.[9] Parents of affected children often report that their child's speech is better at home than during an office visit. Unfortunately, in many situations, both the child's physicians and therapists discount this information. The common explanation for this apparent discrepancy is simply that the family has *learned* how to decipher the child's difficult speech. I had a different view from the start, thanks to two summers of scoring videotapes of adults with a stutter speaking in different research situations. External differences such as fatigue and stress can disrupt the child's speech performance and lead us to overestimate the actual amount of speech impairment. The speech at home is the best indicator of what the brain can do, just as the run, not the walk, reflects the degree of motor recovery. Looking back, this experience was my first exposure to examining the full range of available skills, and it laid the groundwork for my later understanding of *habit hides recovery*.

Finally, in 1966, I travelled all over Ontario as a research assistant to Harvey Stancer, in a project designed to discover if blind women experienced menarche (their first menstrual period) earlier than those with sight. This project gave me further insight into clinical research and led to my getting credit, while still an undergraduate, on a published research paper (under my maiden name, Magee).[10]

This was all exciting and new and led me to believe that research was relatively easy. I had been well trained in experimental design in the psychology department at McGill. As well as a mandatory course in statistics, every course involved a critical appraisal of the published literature and a discussion of how the authors reached their conclusions. We rarely used textbooks (most were notoriously out of date) and instead were given photocopies of actual studies to discuss. All of this training led me to expect well-designed and well-thought-out experiments. So I was totally unprepared to deal with what I learned in the interview of a blind woman who had been born in United States.

Shortly after this woman's birth, she was enrolled in a multicentre, randomized controlled trial (RCT) on the use of oxygen in babies born prematurely. RCTs are widely regarded as the only legitimate and decisive test of treatments in medical circles. These trials involve subjects who are divided at random into groups so that one group is administered treatment and the other, as a "control," is not. Starting in the 1940s, there was an epidemic of retrolental fibroplasia (RLF), a new type of blindness in premature babies. To some, it was clear that this outbreak of blindness coincided with the early use of incubators and high levels of oxygen. Unfortunately, other observational studies seemed to contradict this conclusion. A heated debate took place about the ethics of conducting a research trial on tiny babies, but eventually, the first RCT was done in the mid-1950s. It showed *conclusively* that there was more RLF in the high-oxygen group and less in the restricted-oxygen group. From that time on, oxygen was used on a restricted basis.[11]

The young woman I interviewed had been randomly assigned to the high-oxygen group. As a result, she developed severe RLF and was totally blind. She was alive, but she lived a challenging life and her eyes, besides being sightless, were painful. I walked away from the interview shaken and questioning, as many others had, the ethics of using this type of experimental design in human babies.

Subsequent research studies have examined the effect of different oxygen levels on the incidence of RLF. The goal was to determine the "right" level of oxygen in the blood. After a series of large multicentre randomized controlled trials, studies that have involved thousands of babies and cost millions of dollars, the results are inconclusive: "The clinically appropriate range for oxygen saturation in preterm infants is unknown."[12] Despite the enormous cost and despite having put the health and sight of these babies at risk, studies using the RCT design have failed to determine the exact "best" balance of oxygen for premature infants. You could argue that we are really no further ahead than we were a half-century ago.

Albert Einstein was credited with defining insanity as doing the same thing over and over again in the hope of achieving a different result. I believe it is time to question the dominant theory that the randomized controlled trial is the gold standard for research studies in biomedicine. It may be the best design in some cases, but is it the best design for sorting complex medical problems with multiple interacting variables? In Hebb's department of psychology and four summers of applied research experience, discussions of a research study always started with questions about whether or not the research design was an appropriate one to answer the research question. Currently, in neurorehabilitation, growing numbers of people are questioning the continued adherence of the medical research establishment to just one study design as being the best in all circumstances. It seems there is a growing scientific revolution in this area as well.[13]

———— • ————

I was getting a taste for research—and for clinical neuroscience. Because the majority of students studying medicine at the University of Toronto had gone through a two-year pre-med program while I was earning a four-year degree at McGill, I was one or two years older than most of them, and miles ahead in terms of research experience. My age set me apart and so did my resistance to the prevailing teaching methods, which tended to rely on rote learning and discouraged questions—so very different from Hebb's psychology department at McGill. Plus the school (and the world generally in the 1960s) was suffused with sexism. For example, in my first-year anatomy class, female reproductive organs were discussed openly and in detail, but when testes and penises were described, the 13 women in the class of 169 were made to leave the room for a private tutorial with a female assistant so as not to embarrass the men!

My fourth year in medicine was the first time in the history of the U of T program that students were moved into a clinical rotation as if they were interns, and, if some of the medical staff had had their way, I would have ended up as an orthopedic surgeon. It was because of my height. The notably tall chief of surgery and orthopedics at the Toronto General Hospital spotted me. His senior resident and fellow also topped out at more than six-foot-five. For doubtless good reasons, the chief had decided that a female pediatric orthopedic surgeon would be good for the department. I remember comments about women's delicate hands being more suited to surgery on infants and children. Seeing that I had an A in surgery and was five-foot-ten, which meant that I didn't need to stand on a footstool to assist them in the operating theatre, he all but shanghaied me. I spent months more of my fourth-year rotation in orthopedics and emergency (where I got more exposure to surgery) than I should have done. At the time, I was more interested in pediatrics and had no idea how important a role orthopedic surgeons and their work would play in my understanding of cerebral palsy.

— • —

I started my pediatric residency in the emergency room in the middle of a meningitis epidemic. At the peak of the outbreak, we were doing hundreds of lumbar punctures a month. I became skilled at this delicate procedure and was asked to stay on for a few more weeks. Although the assignment disrupted my rotation, I found that I enjoyed the intensity of the emergency room, just as I had revelled in the camaraderie of the operating theatre. Pediatrics, however, was what I wanted to do.

The Neonatal Intensive Care Unit, when I got to it as a junior resident, was relatively new and considerably expanded the hospital's capacity to deal with seriously sick infants. Making it bigger didn't make it less busy than it had been before, however: precisely because the medical staff were getting better at what they were doing, more premature and low birth-weight babies were flooding in. By 1970 annual neonatal admissions were around 1300 and the NICU was running at 131 percent of capacity. Of those 1300 infants, some 200 were high-risk, weighing in at less than 1500 grams.

I loved it from the start.

I loved the hustle, the teamwork, and the diagnostic challenge posed by babies. They're a special kind of puzzle because they can't tell you what's going on. You have to study them for clues.

When I started my residency, Sick Kids was the only hospital in Ontario with a dedicated NICU, which meant that it accepted tiny premature babies and full-term asphyxiated newborns from all over the province. As a matter of practical necessity, because there was nowhere else to send them, it had a policy of never turning a baby away. This led to sporadic craziness. One nurse recalled an occasion a few years before I got there when the NICU found itself inundated with almost more patients than it could handle. "We had isolettes and equipment plugged into every available outlet on the unit; babies in the nursing station, in the equipment room, the hallways, the fluoroscopy room, admitting and exchange treatment rooms. The rooms had wall-to-wall isolettes."[14] Her words reflected the stress of working there but also the pride the staff took in handling it. We continued to be swamped at times, but the coping attitude never changed.

The hours were ridiculous. To manage the often-over-flowing unit, there was one staff doctor, a research fellow doing clinical service, two senior residents, and two juniors like me on a monthly rotation. We worked twelve-hour shifts (from six in the morning to six at night) every other day and every other weekend. We rotated being on call, which meant that after a mostly sleepless night, you would be working the next day until six the following evening. And once again (I was younger then!) I couldn't get enough of it. My attitude was rewarded and my time in the NICU was extended by a couple of months in both my junior and senior years.

The head of the new department of neonatology was an Englishman, Dr. Paul Swyer, who had been recruited by his predecessor more than a decade before. Swyer was the author of a privately published history whose subtitle, "The Fight for Intact Survival at the Hospital for Sick Children, 1875–2000," reflected the main goal of HSC doctors through-out his tenure—to give preemies a fighting chance to live a normal life. In fact, at Sick Kids and at other hospitals with the same mission, the odds got better over the years. Mortality of infants with a birth weight of less than 1500 grams was a staggering 85 percent when Swyer joined the staff in 1961; by the mid-1970s, the percentage was down to 31 percent—a huge drop.[15] The change was brought about by a number of factors. Better prevention of certain conditions through immunization; improved ventilation, nutrition, and treatments for a variety of illnesses; and the introduction of dedicated transport teams to bring sick infants to the hospital all contributed to a significant reduction in infant mortality. Swyer taught his residents and fellows that survival alone was not enough. He cared deeply about the quality of the child's life beyond survival.

— • —

After completing my general pediatric training I started a neonatal fellowship under the mentorship of Dr. Pam Fitzhardinge. Pam had been recruited by Paul Swyer to run a fully funded Neonatal Follow-up Program to monitor development and evaluate cognition in post–NICU survivors. We did extensive testing and examinations to screen for cerebral palsy as well as visual and hearing loss. The purpose of the clinic was to help us improve medical care, nutrition, and social interaction with parents, but especially to track treatment and neurologic outcomes. We needed to know the quality of their survival.

Brusque and businesslike, Pam wore her hair cut short, and a pair of horn-rimmed glasses gave her a severe appearance that was not altogether misleading. She was an absolutely outstanding neonatologist and we were fortunate to have lured her away from the Children's Hospital in Montreal. Under her direction, one of my tasks in the Follow-up Program was to track patients from their arrival through their first three or four years of life. Every day I wrote on little index cards a summary of what was happening with every high-risk infant in the unit. In a way, I was repeating my experience as a clerk at Women's College Hospital, but with a diligence and purpose that was new. Pam was one of the first to do more than just quantify survival—certainly, she was the first to do this in Toronto. It's hard to get a clinic like that funded these days, which is too bad: what we derived from the follow-up studies in terms of practical knowledge was incalculable. All of us who had a hand in the program ended up better doctors because of it.

Pam set up a protocol that had us assessing our patients at full term or on discharge and again at three, six, nine, twelve, and eighteen months and then at two years. Some children were seen until three to four years of life, depending upon their condition. An independent child psychologist gave the Bayley Scales of Infant Development to all the children at eighteen months corrected age (corrected by taking into account their prematurity). This was a global test to measure motor performance and intelligence. They also had routine examinations by a neuro-ophthalmologist as many of the preterm babies still developed retrolental fibroplasia, which damages the retina at the back of the eye, and some of the full-term babies had cortical visual impairment, which is damage to the occipital lobes of the brain. I saw the effects of blindness on growth and development and I knew, from the early blindness study with Harvey Stancer, more about its long-term impact. We also screened for hearing loss, as deafness too was more common back then. I had a very focused exposure to both normal and abnormal development in babies who were born with a normally developed brain and then suffered some form of perinatal injury, and I learned how this damage had different expressions depending on the presence or absence of the common comorbidities (that is, the associated diseases and conditions) of cognitive delay and speech, vision, or hearing impairments. Pam taught us how to become expert at the early diagnosis of cerebral palsy and cognitive delay, the two most common neurologic problems seen in Neonatal ICU survivors.

Later in my career I would sometimes encounter parents of children with a condition that they had been told was rare. Often I would know immediately what was wrong. The parents would say, "How can you tell? How can you be so sure?" I had examined so many infants in my time at the Hospital for Sick Children, and seen them not just once or twice, but repeatedly over a period of months and years, that I had an enormous store of case histories packed away in the back of my mind. I became expert in the diagnosis and early management of babies and young children with abnormal neurology in the newborn period. It was the best possible training. I owe a lot to Paul Swyer and Pam Fitzhardinge.

three

Evidence of Baby Brain Neuroplasticity

I was still in the first year of my neonatal fellowship when I was given the opportunity to compete for a Mead Johnson workshop for NICU fellows, which was held annually at Marco Island in Florida. That year the theme was brains, and fortunately for me, I was the only fellow in the unit with an abiding interest in the brain. It was a four-day program with lectures in the morning and early evening. All afternoon we had the opportunity to relax and talk with the presenters. Two of the presenters made a lasting impact on me. The first was Domenic Purpura, a developmental anatomist at Mount Sinai Hospital in New York. He taught us how immature baby brains really are. One fact stuck in my mind above all others: the cerebellum of an infant born at full term still contains many immature nerve cells called neuroblasts. These cells continue to divide and migrate and differentiate to form the mature cerebellum—but it takes three to four years for this to happen in humans.

The generally accepted theory of human brain development at this time was very different. Medical schools still taught students that babies were born at term with all of their brain cells for life. What we had at birth was it, the sum total of what we had to work with for all our days on Earth. Looking at this statement now, it seems almost unbelievable, and, in fact, because of my exposure to the neuropsychology department at McGill, I did not believe it. It did not make sense that neurons would not die and regenerate, as did every other cell in the body. It has been estimated that all the cells in your body turn over every two to three years. The ones in your gut do it every few days! What Purpura, in 1975, was teaching about human brains was another example of heretical thought. He showed us slides of immature cerebellums packed full of migrating and dividing neuroblasts. Over the first two years of life, he explained, these neuroblasts continue to move from the deep central areas of the cerebellum to the outer cortical area. Once there, they start to divide into three distinct layers and specialize into the eight different types of cerebellar neurons. Only then could they manage to wire up and start working.

The mature cerebellum helps control rapid fine motor movements, among other things, and it can also serve as backup for damaged gross motor control systems.[1] This means that the ability of a child to button a coat or learn to print is tied to changes in the brain that continue to evolve for as long as four, five, or even six years. When I learned this, in the mid-1970s, it was all new and exciting. With improved measurement techniques, we now know that up to 50 percent of all the neurons (brain cells) in the brain are found in the cerebellum and the majority of them are produced after birth. The late development of the cerebellum in humans and its central importance to how our brains work has only recently become a hot topic in brain research.[2]

The other presenter at the Marco Island workshop whose work impressed me was Jonathan Wigglesworth, an eccentric perinatal pathologist from Hammersmith Hospital in London, England. He set out to challenge the standard thinking about bleeding into the brains of babies who were born prematurely. Bleeding into the brain is one of the most common findings in the brains of premature babies who die. The commonly accepted explanation was that this bleeding was caused by a backup of blood in the veins close to the centre of the brain. Dr. Joseph Volpe, a prominent neonatal neurologist, noted that the terminal vein had a prominent kink, like an abrupt U-turn, just where the bleeding seemed to originate. "This change in the direction of blood flow would be expected to encourage venous stasis, congestion and rupture of the small vessels."[3] In a series of lectures at the workshop, Wigglesworth demonstrated that this theory was plain wrong.[4] His injection studies showed conclusively that "extensive destruction of the subependymal capillary bed occurs without arterial or venous rupture."[5]

So it wasn't kinky veins.

Wigglesworth was able to show that the bleeding so commonly found in preterm baby brains issued not from a kinky terminal vein, but from the immature capillaries in the germinal matrix tissue, next to the central ventricles of the brain. He was actually pretty scathing about the old theory. "Kinkiness is Mother Nature's way of growing both veins and arteries," he told us, "and then they straighten out as the brain grows. There are bloody kinky veins everywhere in the immature baby's brain."

Wigglesworth's injection studies that discounted the "kinky vein" theory directly led to a change in our approach to the prevention of bleeding into the brain of the premature infant. If baby brain bleeds were caused by an anatomic abnormality, as argued by Joseph Volpe and many other neonatal neurologists of the time, then there was not much that you could do about preventing the bleeds until the brain matured. Wigglesworth's discovery that the bleeding issued from the small capillaries emphasized the importance of variations in blood flow, which has led to new ways of thinking about how we treat babies in the NICU.[6] He was yet another heretic challenging established theories.

His ideas about the kinky veins in premature babies were startling, to be sure, but his ideas about the maturation of the brain would have a deep impact on how I would treat children with CP caused by brain damage.

Wigglesworth taught us that an infant's brain changes more between twenty-four and forty-four weeks gestational age than it does from birth to senility. Twenty-four weeks is about the earliest point at which a premature infant has a chance of surviving. The baby is fully formed at this point. It weighs about 700 grams, or a pound and a half, and looks just like a miniature baby. A baby this age could easily fit in the palm of your hand. Forty-four weeks is just after full term. The last trimester or so of pregnancy, between twenty-four and forty-four weeks, is a peak time of baby brain growth and maturation. It's also a time when the brain is vulnerable to different types of injury. And here, I would learn, was the critical point: brain injury to a preterm baby differs greatly from brain injury to a full-term infant, or to an eighteen-month-old toddler. Wigglesworth taught me that the outcome after injury was influenced by the state of maturity of the brain *at the time of damage*. This was an incredibly important insight that later helped me sort the different types and expressions of cerebral palsy into groups determined both by what parts of the brain were damaged and also by what normal, undamaged parts were still to develop as the brain grew and matured.

Wigglesworth's theory about bleeds into the baby brain was totally out of line with orthodox thinking, and it was thrilling to hear him expound it. As soon as I returned from the workshop, I asked my boss, Paul Swyer, to invite him to give a talk in Toronto. Funds were needed and arrangements had to be made to bring him over from England, but Paul agreed that it was worth the trouble.

Wigglesworth came. He talked. He impressed me even more. He was working on the frontiers of neuroscience as it applied to babies. After finishing my pediatric and neonatal training, I wanted to work with him. With endorsements from Drs. Swyer and Fitzhardinge, I applied for and won a two-year Duncan L. Gordon Travelling Fellowship from the HSC Foundation. For the first year, I worked with Jonathan

Wigglesworth in the neonatal pathology section of London's Hammersmith Hospital. My first task was to learn more about neonatal pathology by assisting him in performing autopsies on anywhere from one to ten babies a week and then helping work out their cause of death and other relevant details.

Our partnership flourished. After the first month, he asked me to collaborate with him on a book about baby brain hemorrhages. To his original theories and findings, I was able to contribute a neonatal clinical perspective as well as the knowledge I had acquired in the Follow-Up Clinic with Pam Fitzhardinge and the neuroradiology department with Derek Harwood-Nash in Toronto. Margaret Norman and Dawna Armstrong, both physicians in the pathology department of Sick Kids, had also introduced me to a non-hemorrhagic lesion of baby brains called periventricular leukomalacia, or PVL, a type of ischemic damage found only in the immature brain.[7] Their paper describing this pathologic finding in premature brains had just been published in 1974 and was not yet widely known. By the time our book was written, we changed the title to *Haemorrhage, Ischaemia and the Perinatal Brain* and we published an integrated theory of how both these lesions could occur singly or together as a result of variations in blood flow to vulnerable, rapidly growing areas of the immature brain.[8]

The next year, I became an honorary senior registrar at University College Hospital, also in London, working with

Professor Osmund Reynolds. Before I left Hammersmith, Jonathan took me to dinner at the Royal College of Physicians. He thought I would be interested in the speaker's topic and he wanted me to see the building the college then occupied, as it was historic and quite beautiful. The talk, which was fascinating, was given by Stuart Campbell, a pioneer in the use of ultrasound scans of pregnant women. Ultrasound scans were then a brand new technology. I was intrigued when the speaker showed us a slide of a baby with congenital hydrocephalus, in which there is a build-up of fluid in the brain while the baby is still in the uterus. In this baby, there was a malformation of the brain that led to the build-up of fluid, but it looked on the ultrasound scan just like the hydrocephalus that sometimes develops in a premature baby after a large bleed into the brain. In conversation with him afterwards, I asked Professor Campbell if the ultrasound technique would be useful in my work with babies. He said no, because the bones in the baby's skull would distort the ultrasound waves.

"But that shouldn't be a problem," I said, "if the waves are directed through the fontanel."

This is the "soft spot" on an infant's head where the bone isn't fully formed. It is very large in premature infants. For a moment he was at a loss for words. He almost sputtered. This was something he hadn't considered. Finally he nodded.

"Of course you can," he said.

Luckily for me, the obstetrics department at University College Hospital had just taken possession of a new portable ultrasound machine, but they wanted it for a research project of their own. After a good deal of discussion and pleading, I got access to the machine, but only when others weren't using it, between five in the evening and nine in the morning. This was fine by me. The engineers taught me what I needed to know to operate the machine and I adjusted my hours to make the most of the opportunity. I arrived at work late and stayed even later performing ultrasound scans on as many babies in the unit as I could legitimately get my hands on.

I was in the right place at the right time. I had just spent a year dissecting the brains of babies who had died in the neonatal period, which made it easier for me to figure out what I was seeing on those very crude, early scans. The first study was done with the ultrasound machine directly through those interfering skull bones, as the "head" of the scanning unit was too big to use on the fontanel. Professor Campbell was right—the skull did distort the images and those first ultrasound images were terrible, but they were still clear enough to see when there was a big hemorrhage or early signs of hydrocephalus. Armed with the data I collected that year, my team wrote the first papers that used ultrasound to diagnose baby brain injury in the NICU.[9] Shortly afterwards, the ultrasound industry came up with smaller, lighter scanner heads so that scans through the anterior fontanel became possible.[10] Much better quality cranial ultrasounds are now used routinely in NICUs everywhere. The chief advantage of an ultrasound scan was that it could be done at the bedside and the baby did not need to be sedated.

On my return to Canada, I started at HSC as a staff neonatologist in the NICU and the Neonatal Follow-Up Clinic in

August 1979. Over the next ten years, I worked half the year in the NICU and the other half in Follow-Up while continuing my research on brain injury. When Pam Fitzhardinge left HSC to run the NICU across the street at Mount Sinai Hospital, I became director of the HSC's Neonatal Follow-Up Clinic. I was promoted from assistant to associate professor in pediatrics. Over the next few years, my research work led to cross appointments to the Institute of Biomedical Engineering, the Division of Exercise Sciences, and the School of Graduate Studies at the University of Toronto. I travelled widely to pass on what I knew about ultrasound scans and to present the findings from my ongoing research.

I had become a recognized expert on detecting and assessing the damage that can affect the infant brain. But, like almost everyone involved in neonatal care at the time, my focus was on diagnosis and evaluation. I was learning more about what brain damage looks like and how it leads to dysfunction. The dominant theory at that time, one that was almost universally shared, was that the outcome after brain injury, whatever it was, was inevitable. It couldn't be changed. The best we could do was to try to prevent the damage in the first place. For those babies with an abnormal CT or ultrasound brain scan, we often faced the ethical dilemma of whether or not we should continue full-on care or stand back and let nature take its course. We had endless discussions and debates among the neonatologists and nurses about how to decide when a baby's brain damage was too great to prolong life. It was not an easy problem to solve. Faced with not much to offer in the way of hope for recovery or treatments to help the baby after a brain injury, we all focused our attention primarily on prevention.

———— • ————

From time to time I came upon a case that puzzled me, an infant whose brain damage showed up on a brain scan who either did not develop cerebral palsy or developed only mild symptoms despite an apparently severe injury.

A young intern who was assigned to the Neonatal Follow-Up Clinic brought Andrew to my attention. I had asked him to do the primary examination of a six-month-old baby with an uncomplicated back story. Andrew had been born prematurely and needed careful monitoring, but there had been nothing untoward in his development, no seizures or other signs that would give cause for alarm. He had appeared to be doing well at his three-month examination. I expected nothing more from the intern's report than news that Andrew was still developing well. This was not what I got.

The intern had been with the infant for about fifteen minutes when he rushed into my office, obviously excited, and announced that Andrew had a big problem and that I had to see it for myself. I was dubious but I followed him to Andrew's cubicle, conducted an examination, and found nothing wrong. Andrew seemed normal.

"What's the problem?" I asked.

The intern, pleased with himself, said, "I'll show you!"

He turned down the overhead lights and pressed a flashlight to the baby's head. The result was shocking: one side lit up like a Halloween pumpkin with a candle inside! Half of Andrew's cranium, with the light behind it, emitted an eerie orange glow.

In the days before CT brain scans became widely available, transillumination of the skull was a standard diagnostic procedure done on infants in the first year of life. Examination rooms in the clinic were equipped with a special flashlight fitted with a rubber attachment to ensure good contact with the skull. The flashlight was pressed against the head in a darkened room and switched on. A negative transillumination test of a normal head would show only a dim glow around the head of the flashlight. But if there was an abnormal build-up of fluid where brain tissue was missing, that part of the skull would light up. By the early 1980s we had pretty much abandoned the flashlight test: if we suspected brain damage, we sent the infant for a CT scan. But nobody had told the intern this and his old-fashioned enterprise had turned up a problem. I had thought Andrew was developing normally.

I had him admitted to the neurology ward and asked for a head CT scan. The neurology team looked at him—without the flashlight—and said he was fine. So I wasn't the only one who missed it! They were as shocked as I was when they saw what the intern had found.

Andrew's scan revealed that a massive stroke had affected the middle cerebral artery distribution on the right side of his brain. A large cyst had replaced the damaged tissue. This was the fluid-filled cavity that lit up when the flashlight was held against his head. This damage to his brain had occurred very early in life, probably in the uterus before birth. All the areas responsible for moving and feeling in one side of his body were gone. I still did not understand his "normal" six-month clinical neurologic examination, but armed with the CT scan showing extensive damage to the right side of his brain, I gave his parents my prognosis: I expected him to develop cerebral palsy, specifically a hemiplegia affecting his left arm and leg. I warned that he might also have problems with learning and memory. Virtually half of his brain had been destroyed. At this point, I had never encountered a child with such significant unilateral damage. We got him registered in the local early intervention therapy program and we hoped for the best.

But Andrew had more surprises in store for us. As he grew up and reached early school age, he did not develop left-sided cerebral palsy. Apart from a mild learning disability, his neurologic examination was normal at age seven.

I told a friend, another of my mentors, Bruce Hendrick, about Andrew. At that time, I didn't know that Bruce, a pediatric neurosurgeon, had been among the first to do a therapeutic hemispherectomy removing half of a baby's brain. He wasn't surprised by what I had to say. Andrew, he told me, was recovering as well as his patients who had early hemispherectomies.

Bruce and his colleagues had published a report after performing seven hemispherectomies over a period of a dozen years, the first in 1964.[11] It's not an operation they undertook lightly: his young patients were in a bad way. All suffered from Sturge-Weber syndrome, a rare, progressive (meaning

that it gets worse over time) congenital disorder characterized by a port wine discolouration or birthmark on the face
and neurologic damage from excessive blood vessel growth
in the brain. The birthmark occurs on the same side of the
head as the brain damage. An infant born with Sturge-Weber
syndrome may develop uncontrolled seizures leading to a
progressive hemiplegia affecting the limbs on one side. This
is very different from the typical hemiplegia resulting from
a neonatal brain injury: the child with this problem becomes
more disabled over time. Most of the affected children also
have a severe cognitive impairment that may be worsened
by the heavy doses of medication needed to control the seizures. It's a tough prognosis, one that justifies a creative and,
perhaps, drastic response.

The suggestion that a hemispherectomy might be performed as treatment for Sturge-Weber syndrome was made
at least as early as the 1930s. A South African surgeon, Dr.
Roland Krynauw, reported performing it on a dozen ailing
infants in the 1950s. And by the 1960s, others besides Hendrick were resorting to it. Their results weren't perfect—the
children do not generally emerge from the treatment as good
as new—but the results were remarkable just the same. Of the
seven children operated on at HSC, one was seven years old
when he went under the knife. He was assessed at the outset
as having a subnormal intelligence, and that didn't change,
but his seizures went away completely. The others all had
their hemispherectomies at a much earlier age, between one
and ten months, and while their post-operation experience
varied, all who survived had normal intelligence, leading

Hendrick and his colleagues to conclude that the younger the patient, the higher their eventual IQ. One of the little ones had complications after the operation and did not survive. Another had bilateral damage—damage to both sides of the brain—and continued to have occasional seizures. The others were seizure-free. The degree of physical impairment of the youngest survivors was also strikingly less severe than that of the boy who was operated on when he was older. They could walk with an almost normal stride length and were able to use the weak-side arm and even, to some extent, the hand and fingers. They could manage all this—with just half a brain.[12]

This surgical outcome challenged everything about brain damage that I had been taught in medical school, where the prevailing orthodoxy was built on the concept of brain specificity. Each side of the brain, according to this theory, controlled the opposite side of the body. If one side was removed, the function would be lost. The fact that all the children—even the seven-year-old—walked after having undergone a hemispherectomy clearly demonstrated that when it came to motor function the old rules no longer applied.

—— • ——

Medical specialties don't mix much. We all tend to hang out with our professional peers: my friendship with Bruce Hendrick was a bit out of the ordinary. (For more on this, and the reasons for it, see Chapter 5.) It's even more unusual for any physician to keep up with developments in unrelated fields. But if we pediatricians and neonatologists had been paying more attention to experiments being performed on animals by brain scientists, we might have been less surprised by the outliers we sometimes encountered in our practice. Indeed, if I had made the connection between what I had learned long ago from Donald Hebb and the work I was doing with children, I might have understood the full significance of early maladaptive habits sooner than I did. But in the 1980s, the people doing animal research on the complex workings of the brain and the physicians who treated ailing infants in a clinical setting occupied different worlds. At best, we visited one another, remarked politely on one another's discoveries, and never considered how they might have practical implications for our patients.

But I did pay an occasional visit to that other world.

I audited a graduate-level neuroscience course at Toronto Western Hospital in the early 1980s. In the course we discussed the fascinating work being done mainly with rats in the lab and, less frequently, in longer-term experiments with monkeys. I quickly realized that the young graduate students, who had limited clinical exposure to babies, had no clear idea of the hazards of extrapolating the findings of animal work to humans. I only knew about this problem through my work with Jonathan Wigglesworth. In the book we wrote together, Jonathan contributed a chapter on precisely this subject.[13] In animals and humans, many of the basic science questions about growth and function of the components of a brain are similar. In all species, for example, the way brain cells depolarize and fire is similar. Ditto for the way they wire up into neural networks to form facilitated circuits. Scientists can take bits of brain out of many animal species to see what happens, but baby rats are not baby humans and some of those differences are important.

I met Bryan Kolb, one of the scientists engaged in important animal research, at a neuroplasticity conference. He has a useful ability to translate complicated ideas into simple terms. He is also among the foremost Canadian neuroscientists to have focused his research on the capacity of the brain to grow, change, and adapt to different experiences. He set out as a researcher to discover, for example, what happens inside the brain when it is physically hurt or exposed to different drugs and hormones. How does it change? Can it recover? He was the first to show that stimulants can be used to induce growth of new brain cells, a process called neurogenesis, which until recently was regarded by many scientists as impossible.[14]

Much of Kolb's work has been with rats. In a series of experiments that he wrote up with a colleague, Jo-Anne Tomie, in 1988, he tested the effect of a hemidecortication, which is taking out half the brain and then some. Some of the rats had one hemisphere removed as adults, and a group of younger rats had their surgery at one, five, or ten days of age. Laboratory rats are considered mature adults by six months of age with a lifespan of two to three years or longer in captivity. After they had recovered from surgery, all the rats were put through a series of tests. They'd have to find their way in a maze, walk on a beam, turn, and swim. It was a way to assess their cognitive skills and physical functions. In all the tests the animals with operations done at the early age did better than the ones who had surgery later in life. The conclusion was obvious: young animal brains can recover better than older ones can.

Kolb noticed something else: in the rats that lost one side of their brain, the other side grew bigger. The baby rats grew a significant amount of new brain tissue after losing half their brain. Could this be the case with young children who have had half their brains removed by surgery?

A 2012 review of twenty years of monkey studies also showed that the younger ones did far better after hemispherectomy than the older ones. Younger monkeys did better in a variety of tests, including both motor and visual function, and even in their sensitivity to temperature change and pain. The younger animals also recovered the use of their lower limbs completely after the operation, while older animals struggled. The same review made an intriguing observation about humans: after an early surgery removing half their brain, children can walk nearly perfectly if they get physical training.[15]

In a way, none of this is new. The scientists reviewing the work with monkeys in 2012 were reporting results that were known, at least in a general way, to researchers decades earlier. This is what scientists do: they repeat experiments originally devised by others, but with minor variations, to find out if the results hold up. This, as Kuhn pointed out, is normal science doing its work.[16]

— • —

Sometimes we know more than we know. By this stage of my career, in the late 1980s, I knew about hemispherectomies.

I also knew about a young man who had damage to both sides of his brain and still recovered, which is something that isn't supposed to happen—ever. Conventional wisdom now has it that, in certain circumstances, we can get by if one hemisphere is removed early in life so long as the other side is normal: the undamaged side often has the capacity to take over. But if both hemispheres are damaged, the likelihood of full recovery is essentially nil. And yet there are outliers.

There was an infant treated in the NICU at Hammersmith Hospital, London, who had massive bilateral brain damage. He had lost the equivalent of half a brain in total, but the damage affected both sides—roughly half of each side of the brain was destroyed. And yet, at seventeen months, he was up and walking—doing pretty well. I never saw him, but Jonathan Wigglesworth included his brain scans and a follow-up photo of him up in a book chapter titled "Plasticity of the Developing Brain."[17] It was one more piece of evidence that a human infant can recover, not just from one-sided brain injury, but also—in rare instances—from brain damage to both sides of the brain. It all depends on how much normal brain is left to compensate for the loss.

By the time Jonathan and I were asked to be the editors of the book *Perinatal Brain Lesions*, published in 1989, we could easily pull together experts from many different disciplines to contribute their knowledge to this growing field.[18] The number of scientific and clinical observations that were not explained by the dominant theory that human brain injury was permanent and irreversible was growing, faster in some sub-specialties than others, but they were mounting up. The neurosurgeons and animal researchers led the way, and the wider use of brain scans in the NICU brought neonatologists into the discussion.

four

Baby Brain Neuroplasticity Ignored

M ost of us know the signs that warn of an impending stroke in an adult. Hospital emergency wards have established protocols for dealing with them within hours of the first sign of trouble.[1] There are also best-practice and evidence-informed protocols for recovery. The older men and women who recover from a stroke are no longer thought of as outliers. Thanks in large part to the widespread acceptance of neuroplasticity in the adult medical world, significant recovery of function is something we've come to expect.

We now know that young animals recover from brain injury even better than the adults. And we know that young children subjected to hemispherectomy surgery have an excellent chance of recovering most functions. Is there any logical reason to think that children who have suffered perinatal brain injury, infants from the NICU born prematurely or with significant birth asphyxia, cannot recover as well, if not better than adults with a similar injury?

Every neurosurgeon and most neonatologists know of cases—like the little girl described in the introduction to this book—in which infants or young children with more or less massive brain damage have confounded conventional wisdom by growing up to lead a normal life. Thanks in part to the work of writers such as Norman Doidge and Oliver Sacks, most people are familiar with the concept of neuro-plasticity. It has become routine to accept that the brain can change under certain conditions. But when it comes to children with cerebral palsy, there is less expectation that the brain has plasticity. In order to continue to believe that early human brain injury is permanent and irreversible, we would have to believe that …

Adult animals may recover from brain injury.

Adult humans may recover from brain injury.

Young animals recover better than adult animals.

Young humans do not recover???

This makes no sense at all.

— • —

The philosopher of science mentioned earlier, Thomas Kuhn, noted that scientists (along with the rest of us) tend to ignore observations that don't fit with a prevailing theory. It took a long time, for example, for people to get used to the idea that the Sun doesn't circle the Earth, despite all kinds of evidence that it's the other way round. Something similar happened when researchers first started to report that infants with the kind of brain injury usually associated with cerebral palsy sometimes get better all on their own.

The first study that documented exactly how often our predictions with regard to diagnosing cerebral palsy were wrong was published by Karin Nelson and Jonas Ellenberg, all the way back in 1981. They and their team of researchers didn't have the benefit of CT brain scans or MRIs to assess the presence or absence of brain damage. They tracked the progress of children who had difficulties at birth that were documented by a low Apgar score. This test, which assesses newborn infants on a ten-point checklist of function, is still used in delivery rooms everywhere as a standardized measurement of how the baby is adjusting to life after birth. Nelson and Ellenberg had the children assessed for signs of motor or cognitive handicap at one year and then again at age seven.[2] The results were astonishing: they found that the score was a good way to assess quickly if the baby needed further resuscitation, but "of the children who had Apgar scores of 0 to 3 at ten minutes or later and survived, 80% were free of major handicap at early school age." In other words, 80 percent of the babies with the lowest Apgar scores somehow recovered completely. Baby brains are clearly more resilient than adult brains.

The second part of their study, published a year later, was even more interesting. They examined the records of 37,282 children who had their Apgar scores recorded at birth. Of these, 229 children were diagnosed as having CP at one year.

To be clear, these 229 children were not considered *at risk* of developing cerebral palsy—they were considered to have all the signs and symptoms of definite mild, moderate, or severe forms of this supposedly permanent neurologic problem.

When the seven-year examination was completed, of the 229 who had been diagnosed with cerebral palsy, in 118—almost exactly half—the motor signs of cerebral palsy had resolved. Their CP was gone. The predictions were wrong.

The researchers found that among the children diagnosed with mild CP at one year, 75 percent recovered. Those with moderate signs at one year had a recovery rate of 44 percent, while only one of the most severely affected group recovered.

These results were stunning: either the initial diagnosis was wrong a lot of the time, or the infants had recovered. Nelson and Ellenberg were very careful in their conclusion: "The major practical implication of this study is that, because abnormal motor signs in young children may subsequently normalize, it is appropriate to exercise caution in labeling young children with mild motor disorders, and in predicting future motor impairment."[3] They urged caution in the mild group, where 75 percent recovered, but neglected to mention the 44 percent of moderately involved children who also recovered.

To appreciate how revolutionary this study was, remember what the prevailing view was at the time. It said that baby brain damage was permanent and irreversible and the signs and symptoms of cerebral palsy, once diagnosed, were there for life.

The defenders of the old paradigm found an ingenious way to explain away the 118 toddlers with definite abnormal signs that inconveniently went away. A new condition, transient dystonia, was created to accommodate the new facts. In any population of high-risk infants, this line of thinking went, neurologic abnormalities are relatively common in the first years of life. Problems include muscles that are stiffer than normal and muscles that are weak. In some infants there is alternating stiffness and weakness. The phenomenon of fluctuating tone in this period is called "dystonia." If it goes away by age two years, it's called "transient dystonia." And in those cases where the abnormalities persist past age two years, the diagnosis becomes cerebral palsy.

To this day, many doctors hold off making a diagnosis of CP until a child is at least two, and often three or even four years old. This delay removes all the babies with spontaneous recovery from consideration. As far as the medical community is concerned, these children do not have CP. There are two problems with this approach. First, by not recognizing evidence of early brain recovery, parents are given an unnecessarily hopeless prognosis for their child. Second, by holding off on the diagnosis of cerebral palsy, no treatment is recommended, apart perhaps from a bit of stretching. Parents are told to watch and wait. Some lucky ones may be referred to an early intervention program, but without a definite diagnosis of cerebral palsy, specific cerebral palsy therapies that are routine in the older child are not made available to the toddler.

— • —

Nelson and Ellenberg were not the only ones whose work was raising questions about the permanent nature of brain damage in infants. CT scanning was a new technology in the mid-1970s, and scanners were fairly rare. We had one at the Hospital for Sick Children, but it was five floors down at the other end of the hospital. Not all preterm infants made that journey. We took only the babies who had clinical signs of brain damage, such as a bulging fontanelle or a sudden drop in blood pressure. It was a self-fulfilling prophecy. Most often we were right and the scan showed a bleed into the brain, and if one of these babies died, I would attend the autopsy to make sure that what we had seen on the scan was really there.

Lu-Ann Papile, a researcher at the University of New Mexico, was smart enough to spot the flaw in our procedure. That is, because we were scanning only the infants in whom we expected to see a bleed, we weren't necessarily identifying all the bleeds in our hospital's population of premature infants. We had a first-class selection bias going that ensured that only the sickest babies were scanned. She obtained permission and money to do a population study, meaning that she ran a CT scan on every premature baby with a birth weight equal to or less than 1500 grams who came into her intensive care unit, whether or not the baby had signs of neurologic damage. What she discovered was surprising.

There were forty-six infants in her study, and out of the forty-six, twenty, or 43 percent, showed evidence of cranial intraventricular hemorrhage—a bleed.[4] This was startling in itself: she was finding far more bleeds than anyone expected. Even more surprising was this finding: "Their study indicated that the classic clinical signs of intraventricular hemorrhage were not always associated with hemorrhage into the brain and that 'silent' events could be of a major size."[5] In other words, you could have a bleed in the brain without any of the signs and symptoms that were commonly associated with a bleed into the brain of a newborn infant. This was a big new finding. Up until this study was published, neonatologists and neurologists were sure that a major bleed into the brain was always associated with defined clinical signs of deterioration. Turns out we were all wrong!

The next question was, What did these brain bleeds mean for the baby? Papile and her colleagues first established a scale to measure the extent of the damage indicated by the scans, ranking the lesions from minor (Grade I) to major (Grade IV).[6] This scale has stood the test of time and is still widely used today. In a subsequent study, they assessed the risk of the babies developing CP after a bleed into the brain. They found that the small Grade I and II bleeds carried a low risk of cerebral palsy: only 9 percent of the infants with a Grade I and 11 percent of those with a Grade II bleed went on to develop CP. More significantly, two of the infants with a Grade III bleed, and two with a Grade IV, recovered completely and turned out to be normal. One of the two children with a Grade III bleed and hydrocephalus (a build-up of fluid on the brain) was also normal at follow-up examination.[7] That was the second big news finding: even a serious bleed in the brain did not necessarily cause long-term damage.

— • —

Most physicians still couldn't accept that so many CP patients in the Nelson and Ellenberg study got better on their own. It was easier to conclude that some doctors had made a mistake and were over-diagnosing the condition; they were just too quick to see something wrong. If that was the case, then doctors got it wrong over half the time. That was a disturbingly high error rate, but for those who clung to the traditional view of permanent early brain damage, the explanation of over-diagnosis aligned with the prevailing view despite the growing evidence that an extraordinary number of babies with early signs of brain damage were recovering completely on their own.

The emergence of CT scans as a diagnostic tool complicated matters. Theoretically, the new technology promised to deliver greater precision in the detection of brain hemorrhage. As mentioned, when the first unit came to HSC, we were unable for purely practical reasons to use it for all fragile newborns. Only the sickest babies were taken down to the radiology department and, not unnaturally, we found what we expected to see. When LuAnn Papile found that a significant proportion of infants had a small bleed and even some very large bleeds that occurred "silently," without any clinical signs of deterioration or subsequent cerebral palsy, her critics, still in denial, suggested that physicians must somehow have missed signs of damage in their examinations. Neurologist Dr. Joseph Volpe wrote,

> *It is startling and disturbing that the large majority of the surviving infants with periventricular hemorrhage*

observed by Papile et al.[8] were said to be free *of clinical signs referable to the lesion. We would suggest that the reader not accept the notion that major periventricular hemorrhage in the premature is a clinically silent event, but rather accept the challenge to look much more closely at the neurologic signs in such infants.[9]*

In other words, there was no such thing as a "silent" bleed in the brain, the critics said. The bleed had caused damage; doctors like Papile just hadn't detected it. Everything was wrong, apparently, except the conventional explanation of the condition.

The four infants with a major Grade III or IV bleed who recovered with no sign of cerebral palsy were largely ignored. In the NICU, we also saw occasional outliers who recovered, but the evidence of these recoveries from a major brain injury somehow did not filter out to the cerebral palsy experts, who still maintained that baby brain injury was permanent and irreversible.

Further studies have confirmed Papile's observation that infants can have very significant abnormalities on neonatal brain scans yet be considered normal at follow-up, but you have to really look for these results. I found some fascinating data in a paper from the Netherlands that investigated the neurodevelopmental outcome of babies born before or at thirty-five weeks gestation who had big bleeds in the neonatal period.[10] Of the original 214 babies with a big bleed, 144 (67 percent) survived. Some 86 percent of the infants with a Grade III bleed had a normal cognitive outcome and were free of any signs of CP. Among the infants with the very worst Grade IV bleed, nearly half had normal brain function and did not have CP. As the authors put it, "our long-term outcome was better than reported earlier."[11] These results are astounding. Currently when a baby in a NICU has a major bleed, most parents are not given anything like these odds of intact survival.

After a major bleed into the brain, some children somehow avoid developing cerebral palsy. They recover, a clear sign of neuroplasticity at work in a baby brain. Yet the ability of the baby brain to change and heal has not yet been widely incorporated into the standard therapy for most children with CP.

— • —

Cerebral palsy is the most common motor disability of childhood, with roughly one new case diagnosed every hour in the United States.[12] William John Little first described what we now know as cerebral palsy in the late nineteenth century. Little's disease, as he saw it, was characterized by a group of orthopedic deformities that he traced to brain injury at birth. Little, along with his contemporaries, documented the condition's widespread effects, which included spasticity, deformity, and mental retardation, for none of which they saw any hope of a cure. William Osler enlarged upon the possible causes of what he was the first to call cerebral palsy in 1888. Besides a variety of traumas suffered at birth (head injury, forceps delivery, and difficult labour), he included among possible causes maternal alcohol consumption, convulsions, syphilis, and embolism from bacterial endocarditis. Like Little, he saw no prospect of recovery. It was a sentence for life.

The worst cases died young. When I was a neonatal resident at the Hospital for Sick Children in the early 1970s, I was told that 50 percent of patients with seizures, swallowing difficulties, and spastic quadriplegia would die in their first year and the rest would be dead before they were ten. They would succumb to aspiration pneumonia, untreated seizures, bedsores, or urinary tract infections.[13] In the 1960s, over 60 percent of neonatal survivors with cerebral palsy would be rated IV or V on the Gross Motor Function Classification System (GMFCS), a standardized assessment of function now widely used to classify severity in children with CP, in which I is mild and V is most severe. Severe perinatal asphyxia at all stages of gestation was much more common in those early days. Prior to dedicated neonatal transport teams, the babies would arrive at HSC in terrible shape.

The other major cause of severe CP was kernicterus, the medical term for a severe form of jaundice caused by rhesus incompatibility between the mother's and the baby's blood. These babies were born with rapidly progressing jaundice, and our treatments, while heroic, in many cases failed to prevent brain damage, which resulted in a severe form of athetoid quadriplegia. Children with athetosis have frequent, uncontrolled movements of the face, arms, and legs that make speaking clearly, eating, or walking difficult. None of the available treatments seemed to improve this type of cerebral palsy, and the failure of rehabilitation to get positive results might have been part of what convinced many physicians that effective treatment for cerebral palsy was limited. But rhesus incompatibility has virtually disappeared in high-income countries thanks to preventive treatment of the Rh-negative mother. Today the severity statistics for children with cerebral palsy have been turned upside down: 80 to 85 percent of children have mild to moderate impairments, scoring at Level I, II, or III on standardized scales of function.[14] Of this group, approximately 60 percent are able to walk independently. Children with cerebral palsy have a near-normal life expectancy, with early death occurring only in the small number of very severely involved children. New best practices in obstetric and perinatal care have made a huge contribution to an improved quality of survival. Improvements throughout the perinatal field have resulted in better function in survivors.

But one thing hasn't changed. The official understanding of cerebral palsy's cause, characteristics, and natural history and the functional outlook for surviving patients are much the same now as they were in the middle of the past century. William John Little thought Little's disease was a life sentence and most pediatricians still agree. Indeed, it's official: from the cerebral palsy information page of the National Institute of Neurological Disorders and Stroke: "The term cerebral palsy refers to any one of a number of neurological disorders that appear in infancy or early childhood and *permanently* affect body movement and muscle coordination."[15]

Doctors are doers: their mission is to help people overcome their illnesses, ailments, and disabilities. But our understanding of cerebral palsy—the way it is defined by the institutions charged with marshalling information about the condition—virtually enforces a hands-off, wait-and-see approach. Adults recover from stroke. There are children living a full life with half a brain. But when it comes to infants who have suffered a perinatal brain injury, the conventional view does not support early treatment to provide the same hope of recovery.

— • —

Why would anyone assume that children lack the resilience we willingly attribute to adults, let alone rats and primates? I believe that it is time to not just document good outcomes but also start to study the outliers, like the babies who myste-riously recovered from a major brain bleed. What made these lucky babies different? What can we learn by studying the children with a good outcome? All neonatologists know of some babies who recover from significant brain injuries, and every experienced therapist has seen children with CP who have exceeded their expectations of recovery. It is time for a new way of thinking about recovery that takes into account the amazing power of young children's brains to regrow, repair, reorganize, and reallocate brain real estate to create function. Why would we think that a child with CP has no chance of learning to walk with a normal gait, grasp a pencil with the weak-side hand, or speak clearly enough to be easily under-stood? Baby brains have neuroplasticity and we need to learn how to translate that fact into better treatment interventions.

I was chatting not that long ago with a pediatric neuro-surgeon, Justin Brown, at a medical conference. How strange it is that many people in the pediatric neurorehabilitation world still don't believe that baby brains get better, I said. I pointed to the kids who did so well after hemispherectomy surgery, which removed a big part of their brain. Wasn't that the ultimate proof of baby brain recovery?

He stopped me. "What do you mean? Everybody knows about hemispherectomies."

"Well, no, they don't," I said. Most people taking care of sick babies didn't know that a child could be normal after losing half of his brain in surgery.

Justin looked surprised. "But that's why I went into neurosurgery."

Justin's understanding of the brain and his approach to its diseases and disorders were formed by his training in a different medical specialty than those physicians who special-ized in cerebral palsy. It is perhaps no coincidence that part of Justin's neurosurgery training was with my friend Bruce Hendrick at HSC. His surprise gives a clue to the factors that shape the way we approach our work. It tells us something about how doctors think.

five

How Doctors Think

While I was working in the NICU and the Follow-Up Clinic at the Hospital for Sick Children, I became increasingly convinced that the evidence was clear: we should adopt a more optimistic outlook and certainly start treatment early if we thought babies were at risk of developing cerebral palsy. Yet I ran into a lot of skeptics, and I found myself repeatedly being drawn into conflict with colleagues. I was not, I confess, overly tolerant. For the most part, I looked on my critics as stubborn defenders of the past.

In this period, I had a few brief meetings with Ursula Franklin, a research physicist at the University of Toronto and the first female professor in the engineering department. It was Franklin who first told me about Thomas Kuhn's book *The Structure of Scientific Revolutions*.[1] Kuhn, she said, would help "Teflon coat" me against the negativity and forces of

conformity, then so prevalent in university and medical communities. She said we could learn *how to do* science in our
research or specialty training, but a Ph.D. or a sub-specialty
in a field of medicine would not teach us *how to think* of
new questions to be answered. Franklin was a change artist
who encouraged me to keep pushing for change in the care
of babies.

Kuhn described how science works—and why it is so
resistant to change. Once a theory has gained widespread
acceptance, scientists mostly engage in a process Kuhn calls
"mopping up." The term is not meant to be disparaging: the
repeated testing of a theory to make sure it's sound was the
legitimate business of science. If it's less glamorous merely
to confirm and refine, we only know if the theories are sound
after they have been thoroughly examined.

Kuhn defined this work as normal science.

If a particular experiment falls short in further studies,
the question most likely to be asked is not, Has the theory
failed? But rather, What is wrong with the experiment? Only
when a large number of trials produce results that under-
mine the theory—trials that are shown to be procedurally
unimpeachable—is the theory likely to be challenged and
ultimately changed.

Kuhn describes a process of change that can be broken
down into phases. In the first phase, a consensus forms with
respect to a paradigm. In the second, normal science sets
about exploring the paradigm's implications. In the third,
the discovery of anomalies that don't fit the theory provokes
a crisis. The fourth marks the revolution in which the old

paradigm is re-examined and ultimately replaced by something new.

The old theory doesn't die without a fight. Of the mopping-up operations that characterize normal science, Kuhn writes:

> *Closely examined, whether historically or in the contemporary laboratory, that enterprise seems an attempt to force nature into the preformed and relatively inflexible box that the paradigm supplies.* No part of the aim of normal science is to call forth new sorts of phenomena; *indeed those that will not fit the box are often not seen at all. Nor do scientists normally aim to invent new theories, and they are often intolerant of those invented by others. Instead, normal-scientific research is directed to the articulation of those phenomena and theories that the paradigm already supplies.*[2]

The old theory, or paradigm, with respect to brain growth and recovery depended upon the assumption that the infant brain develops with a large but ultimately limited number of brain cells and a fixed structure. Damage, when it occurs, is permanent. Normal science, within this theory, consists of making whatever adjustments to the existing, damaged structure that are possible. Braces, medication, various therapies, or surgical interventions, according to this interpretation of the disorder, alter the body functions without changing the brain. The notion that the brain can reinvent itself by growing new cells or developing new pathways is alien to this way of thinking. As a result, there is a limit to what can be reasonably hoped for under this paradigm. And anyone who says otherwise is apt to be ignored or disparaged.

After reading Kuhn's book, I felt better. I realized that I was living in the third stage of change where new observations—the outliers—were starting to provoke a crisis. I was one of many scientists and physicians who were challenging the accepted wisdom of this field of medicine, and the workers in normal science were not happy.

———— • ————

Looking back, there are two books that I wish had been published earlier: *Mindset*, by Carol Dweck, and *How Doctors Think*, by Jerome Groopman. Both address the importance of the underlying, often unconscious assumptions we all bring to our work. It would have been enormously helpful to me to know then what I know now. In my career, what I believe to be true has changed with time, experience, and new knowledge. These two books explain that there are both inner and outer forms of resistance to this change.

Carol Dweck's book, *Mindset*, was published in 2007, but I read it only five or six years ago at the suggestion of one of my patients.[3] Dweck, a brilliant psychologist, has spent her career studying the power of established ways of thinking. She starts with a new look at the issue of nature versus nurture with respect to intelligence. People with a fixed mindset believe that intelligence is an inherited trait. A derivative belief is that intelligence can be accurately measured by a single, one-time IQ test and the results of that test can be used to predict a child's academic future. In contrast, people with a growth mindset believe that intelligence, like all human traits, is best thought of as a potential. As Dweck puts it, "potential is someone's capacity to develop their skills with effort over time." She has talked about the power of the word "yet" when added to a child's description of progress in solving a problem. A child struggling with math might say, with finality, "I can't do math," reflecting a fixed mindset. Dweck teaches the child to say, "I can't do math, yet." That one little word transforms a fixed approach to problem solving to a growth approach and so opens up a world of possibility. I now routinely teach children struggling with a motor skill to say, "I can't do it, yet." I reject the idea that this is false hope. Rather, I believe this is an accurate description of the current state of affairs. The first statement closes off all options; the second opens them to the possibility of improvement over time.

An underlying belief that baby brain damage is permanent and irreversible is compatible with a fixed mindset. People with a growth mindset would not be comfortable accepting a child's level of neurologic impairment as a fixed trait, and modern neuroscience thinking would be on their side. Neuroplasticity is a game changer for the rehabilitation world, and it demands a radical shift in our approach to rehabilitation and our expectations for recovery. It means, at the very least, being more open to observations that deviate from norms that have been accepted for years.

Many years ago, I was teaching a course on brain injury to a group of pediatric physical and occupational therapists at the Rehabilitation Institute of Chicago. When I presented the excellent outcomes achieved in some children treated by an early hemispherectomy, the audience had difficulty accepting what I had to say. Could they really both walk and talk after this drastic surgery? I saw doubtful expressions on the faces of members of the audience and I felt them losing interest. Some actually shook their heads. They had been taught nothing about these neurosurgical procedures in the course of their training and it was hard for them to accept my evidence.

It wasn't until after the coffee break that they saw the light. The physician hosting the course brought in a young girl who'd had surgery to treat Rasmussen's encephalitis. Just like the little girl described in the introduction, this child had experienced a sudden onset of severe seizures in a previously normal brain. She had undergone an anatomic hemispherectomy: the right hemisphere of her brain had been surgically removed just weeks earlier. Yet she walked into the lecture room with only a mild limp and demonstrated good functional use of her left hand. It was a terrific demonstration of the effectiveness of the procedure. It also brought about an immediate change in the atmosphere in the room. I realized later that this was a case of growth-mindset conversion—at least with respect to hemispherectomy.

— • —

When I read Jerome Groopman's book, I felt empowered. He explained that there are good reasons why physicians variously ignore, deny, ingeniously explain away, or fail to act on evidence that falls outside the conventional framework. Some of these reasons have to do with the way our brains work—not just physicians' brains, but everyone's. Some reasons are structural, having to do with the way medicine is organized. Still others derive from the conventions of science itself.

In *How Doctors Think*, Groopman, a Harvard-based cancer specialist and regular contributor to *The New Yorker* magazine, explores a multitude of habits and fallacies that may influence a doctor's interpretation of a case.[4] I have mentioned earlier the way we picked the sickest infants for CT scans in the expectation of finding brain damage. This was a prime example of selection bias, just one of the many types of unconscious biases that we all bring to our work. It wasn't the only time I made this type of mistake.

I was a resident at the hospital when I wrote an article intended to draw attention to a situational bias error made by others. I had noticed a baby in the NICU with an abnormal cry, and the staff doctor on service said he had read that this was associated with an increased risk of a congenital heart problem. Douglas Pickering, the cardiac fellow, found nothing wrong with the baby's heart. This was confusing. Then we read the original paper. The authors had noticed a high incidence of asymmetric cry in the children they treated and concluded that there was a link between the cry and cardiac problems. They named this cardiofacial syndrome.[5] But it seemed obvious to us that their results were skewed because they were cardiologists and *all* their patients had a problem with their heart. Pickering and I got permission to undertake a survey. I took a picture of the baby crying to demonstrate the abnormal cry and posted it in wards throughout the hospital.

Our paper, published in the *Journal of Paediatrics* in 1972,[6] found that children with the asymmetric cry could have a wide variety of congenital issues, with or without a cardiac lesion. Some were normal. Which was fine as far as it went. Unfortunately, we made the same mistake as the cardiologists. We also failed to take into account the dangers of a situational bias. Within a year, our mistake was brought home to us.

A neonatologist in Israel, Max Perlman (who later became a colleague of mine in the NICU in Toronto), conducted a study involving 6360 otherwise normal babies in a general population of newborns and found a very low association—just 4.9 percent—between the asymmetric cry and other congenital anomalies.[7] Of course, our sample had showed a higher ratio of children with problems (77 percent): it was drawn entirely from a hospital setting!

— • —

Physicians' biases, and the errors and tendencies to which they're susceptible, may have little effect in the long run: the system has built-in safety measures, and patients themselves play an essential role in managing their health. But sometimes the mistakes are consequential. Groopman points to the case of a patient who had a long history of being treated for anorexia and bulimia (related eating disorders) complicated by irritable bowel syndrome. Her complaints of symptoms that pointed in a different direction were discounted by a number of physicians until, at last, one who was uninfluenced by the previous diagnoses started his examination with a comprehensive history from the first time she felt unwell and correctly diagnosed and treated her celiac disease. In this instance, the last physician's insight not only gave the patient relief from a miserable condition, but it may also have saved her life. In medicine, as it is practised now, there is little opportunity to do a comprehensive history, especially when that history is a lifelong story of a chronic problem like cerebral palsy. As a medical student I was taught that 90 to 95 percent of a correct diagnosis was in the history. It is hard to ask the questions in a ten- to fifteen-minute office visit.

In the summers when I worked at Women's College Hospital with Walter Hannah and spent all those hours poring over patients' charts and, again, when I was following patients' progress and filling out index cards at the Hospital for Sick Children's NICU and Neonatal Follow-Up Clinic, I saw repeatedly how patients' histories were framed, the notes of one attending physician or nurse reiterating and reinforcing the observations of others, without taking into account contradictory data or taking a new look at what was going on with the patient in the bed.

We build routines to protect our patients and ourselves, to make sure that appropriate steps—tests, medications, and procedures—are employed. But sometimes routine can blind us. We are all guilty at one time or another of sticking to familiar paths. The customary way of doing things in the case of Andrew meant relying on a CT scan rather than on an outdated technique—holding a flashlight to his head—with the result that the boy's brain damage was almost missed by a normal clinical examination. Opening our eyes to the unexpected often takes time and experience. Groopman provides in the epilogue to his book a short but informative outline of how best to work through some potential cognitive issues with your doctor when faced with a diagnostic challenge.[8] I consider this book an important read for all patients and acknowledge that it would have helped me to be a better doctor if I had read it earlier.

— • —

The way medicine is organized also plays a part in keeping physicians from accurately assessing new developments and altering their practice to exploit new discoveries in their own and related fields. All patients are aware that different branches of medicine have become highly specialized, but I suspect that not everyone understands how comprehensively the disciplines are divided. We shouldn't be surprised, however: we all accept that lawyers are trained in different specialties. We would not use a real estate lawyer to organize a complicated merger or the acquisition of a large business. Lawyers may be competent in their defined area, but knowledge, especially new knowledge, is segmented and hard to access. The same is true in medicine. Specialists in cerebral palsy treatment have a quite different view of neuroplasticity than do pediatric neurosurgeons. Even pediatricians, although they also work with small children, may have little grasp of recent developments in neonatology. We attend different professional conferences. We subscribe to different medical journals. Our daily routine, the patients we see, the disorders we treat, and the medications we prescribe all are different. We are a multitude of solitudes, communicating, if at all, through referrals and notes on charts.

It's not because we're indifferent to one another's work that we pay so little attention. It's because we're swamped. David Sackett at McMaster University, long regarded as a leader in evidence-based medicine, was one of the first to draw attention to the problem of information overload in medicine. Twenty years ago, he said, just to keep up with developments in internal medicine, a doctor would have to read seventeen articles a day, every day of the year.[9] At the same time, he found that newly graduated doctors typically devoted zero hours to professional reading, while senior consultants put in an average of thirty minutes a day, with 40 percent reading nothing. There was a lot to keep up with then. There's even more now. A recent editorial underlines the challenge you'd face if you happened to be training to be a cardiac imager. (These are radiologists and cardiologists who evaluate stress tests and angiography to look for blocked cardiac arteries, and so on.) As a student, to get totally up-to-date, you'd have to read forty papers a day, five days a week, a task the writer estimated would take eleven years. But by the time you were caught up, you would be seriously behind because, in the time you had spent reading, another 82,000 papers would have been published—which would take you another eight years to read.[10] The plain fact is that science is manufacturing new findings at a faster rate than anyone can absorb. It's literally impossible to keep up.

The pressures of work combined with the unavoidable segregation into professional silos go a long way towards explaining how developments in one area are unnoticed in another. And then there's an additional factor: the march of science is more like a guerrilla operation than a set-piece manoeuvre. There are many more soldiers scouring the underbrush than field marshals with authority to change strategy. Old strategies and old paradigms have a life of their own.

— • —

The recognition that motor skills develop over time and that as the brain grows it can find alternative pathways to compensate for losses was still in my future for much of the time I was working at the Hospital for Sick Children. I was still stuck in the old way of thinking about early childhood rehabilitation. I knew about neuroplasticity and recognized (as had others) that some outliers recovered well. I knew about hemispherectomy surgery and recognized that the old belief that all our brain functions are rigidly specialized to specific areas of the brain was wrong. I had documented unexpected change in children with cerebral palsy in the Neonatal Follow-Up Clinic, but I was still trying to find ways to prevent the occurrence of damage, instead of trying to make it better. I wasn't alone. To this day, I am aware of no systematic study of babies who recover spontaneously from perinatal brain injury, nor any thorough attempt to explain why it happens in some babies but not others.

But still, for me, the anomalies were piling up. The case of Michelle set me on a path that led from abstract study to action and a new approach to treatment and recovery.

six

Use It or Lose It

first met Michelle, the baby who would cause me to transform my treatment of early brain injury, by fluke. It was on
a cold night in December 1982, and I wasn't even on call. The
neonatologist who was supposed to be on duty was struck
down by a bout of diarrhea, and I was summoned to take his
place. The call came from the Neonatal Intensive Care Unit
because the infant who had just been admitted was in a bad
way. I grumbled at being woken in the night but threw on
some clothes and made my way to the hospital.

What happened then, and in the years that followed,
would change the way I understood injuries to the brain,
spinal cord, and nerves—and the way I began to treat them.

Michelle had a forceps delivery that had gone wrong.
The instrument, essentially a pair of steel tongs, is used to
assist an awkward presentation or stalled labour. In this case

we worked out pretty quickly that she had been delivered by a forceps rotation. This is a procedure in which the physician first places forceps around the head to help the baby come out. In this case, the baby's head was stuck. It needed to be turned and then assisted out. Normally the procedure works without a problem, but this time it didn't. This was our opinion at the time, but in the court case that followed, it was ruled that the forceps did not cause the injury.

When Michelle was transferred to the Neonatal ICU, she wasn't moving from the neck down and was unable to breathe without mechanical assistance. Once her condition was stabilized, a test was done in which dye was injected into the spinal cord. The X-ray confirmed what we expected to see: the dye stopped high up, at the second and third vertebrae. This was interpreted as evidence of a complete spinal cord rupture. Her life expectancy was limited.[1]

Although the spinal cord was apparently severed, most of Michelle's brain was undamaged. Her eyes were open and alert and she could cry like any other newborn. She was a real little person. This made the outlook, which was tough under any circumstances, that much harder to contemplate.

In the early days, we all thought it would be better to let her go, if there was no sign of her improving. But we all agreed we had to keep going until we could be sure of the degree of damage. The body goes into shock after a major spinal cord injury. It's like the mechanism that kicks in when the brain is badly hurt and the patient goes into a coma. The whole system goes offline so that other body parts require less oxygen and the brain can go about the job of self-healing.

The shock that follows an injury to the spinal cord can wear off in a couple of weeks or linger for as long as six months. Michelle was stable on a ventilator to breathe for her, and we waited to see if there would be any recovery.

— • —

Michelle had been in the NICU for ten days when a nurse stopped me in the hall.

"Her finger moved," she said.

"What?"

"Her index finger. I saw it move."

I didn't doubt the nurse's report but still, it took me by surprise. If it was really a sign of recovery, it could change everything. There were actually a couple of possible explanations for what she had seen. The movement could have been reflexive, nothing more than a nerve impulse unconnected to the brain causing an incidental muscle spasm. It might have meant nothing.

The other explanation was more hopeful.

The movement the nurse had observed could be an indication that, while Michelle's body was still in deep recovery mode, the spinal cord was not, after all, completely severed.

So we waited and watched and in the next few days there were more tiny movements. Nothing to write home about, but other people, not just the first nurse who reported it, saw them.

And while we waited, the neurologist, the neurosurgeon, the other neonatologists, and I argued about what it meant. Those discussions got pretty heated. Some, including the neurologist, thought the movement was reflexive spinal cord activity and didn't change the initial diagnosis. Others were more positive. I sided with the optimists. But until her body fully emerged from its shock-induced semi-slumber, nothing was known for sure.

Michelle was alert and responsive but chronically ventilated. She could not cough well, which meant she needed frequent suctioning. All of these procedures were painful. We did everything we could to ease her discomfort. At one point, I stumbled on an old negative-pressure ventilator in the basement. This was a big pressurized metal pod, the kind that used to be called an iron lung, into which the patient was inserted, leaving only the head sticking out. They hadn't been used since the 1950s, at the time of the last polio epidemic, and I had to find an engineer to put it back together. I thought if we could get it to work, we'd be able to remove the tube that was damaging Michelle's throat. It didn't work out and she had a tracheotomy tube inserted in her neck to connect to the ventilator. She had continued to show small improvements in her movements, but it was pretty clear she would be chronically ventilated and remain in the hospital.

———— ❖ ————

When Michelle was about a year old, we moved her from the NICU to a newly created chronic ventilator room on a neighbouring ward. There, at least, she would be in a place where night and day were different and the atmosphere was quiet.

And that's where Michelle stayed, becoming a permanent resident. Everyone on the floor got to know her. She was a cute, smart, blond and bright-eyed little girl. Once she learned to speak, she was a little chatterbox. She became a fixture on the ward. Every day she would be strapped into a supportive wheelchair that was rigged out to accommodate a portable ventilator and her suction equipment. After a while, the nurses started to think of her as their own, because they were around her so much and responsible for her well-being.

Her mother, Lyn, was an active participant in her care and a strong advocate for anything she thought would help her child.

"After about three years at Sick Kids, it started to look a lot better," Lyn said. "She was actually communicating. They gave her a talking tracheotomy so she could talk more easily. She was in a unit with other kids who were also trached and on machines. She was starting to come off the ventilator for short periods."

After Michelle moved out of the NICU, I saw her from time to time if she ran into a serious problem. Then, when she was five, her mother came to see me: "You have to do something," Lyn said. "Michelle is moving."

I went to see Michelle during her regular rehab session. The session I watched was with her OT. The therapist was working on supported sitting in the hope that she could get Michelle to start to use her hands in a purposeful way. It appeared to me that she wasn't having a lot of luck but I stayed and watched. When they put her flat on her belly, on a mat, she couldn't really push herself all the way up into a crawling position, as a child who was able-bodied would have done, but she could squiggle and slide in a sort of commando crawl. Think of soldiers crawling under barbed wire. It took her about twenty minutes to wriggle from one side of the mat to the other. At this point, I really wondered what I had done in keeping this little girl alive. She was living in an acute care hospital, with no real expectation of ever leaving. I was the NICU representative on the hospital's ethics committee and tough questions were asked at every meeting. But I had never faced a situation like this. I couldn't stop thinking about her and her dismal future.

And then I realized something. I saw that when she slowly struggled across the therapy mat, every single muscle in her body was actually moving. The left side moved less than the right side, but both sides were moving. It took several days for the significance to sink in. If everything moved, then her spinal cord injury was definitely incomplete. She was now old enough to want to move. She had the brain, spinal cord, nerve, muscle connection, and the will to move and explore her world. The biggest problem, then, was muscle weakness, or disuse muscle atrophy, as the doctors call it. Then the thought occurred to me: if only she had more strength, maybe she could learn to move better.

— • —

The original idea of using electrical stimulation to strengthen Michelle's muscles came from her father, who had used Russian stimulation, or neuromuscular electrical stimulation

(NMES) as it was called in North America, to build muscle mass. It was a new concept and not all therapists were using it.[2] I was a bit familiar with this technique because not long before this, I had injured my knee playing tennis and my physical therapist had used NMES on my quadriceps to strengthen the muscle and aid my recovery. Russian sports scientists had invented it in the 1960s and had been using it with their athletes for years. I thought it might be worth trying on Michelle, that it might give her the boost she needed to start moving independently.

First I talked with her parents and then, because the idea was a new way of treating children and I did not know what to expect in Michelle's case, I took the proposed plan of action to the hospital's ethics panel. The theory I sketched out in my application was that Michelle had suffered a major trauma to her spinal cord at birth—there wasn't any argument about this—and the trauma had precipitated a prolonged period of spinal shock. As a result, other than a few finger movements, she hadn't really attempted to move her body until she was about six months old. Now at five years of age, she could wiggle a bit across a mat and sit with a lot of support, but she did not have independent ability to do anything for herself. She could not even move her arms into a useful position to use her hands.

The theory I proposed was that during the initial period of immobility her muscles got weaker and weaker. As the spinal shock resolved and she tried to move, she lacked the strength to do it. Looking at her function now, I knew the muscles were connected to the nervous system, because she was capable of moving a little bit, but the muscles were not strong enough to move her against the force of gravity. Some of the pathways from her brain through her injured spinal cord were intact. Electrical stimulation was a technology that had been shown to help strengthen weak muscles. It worked for adults. It was reasonable to think that it would work for children too.

The ethics panel told me to go ahead.

NMES uses a relatively high-intensity electrical current that is passed through the muscle for a brief period of time. I attached the electrodes to Michelle's rear chest and abdomen when we first tried it because I thought it might help to strengthen her respiratory muscles and diaphragm—to get her lungs working independently. I adjusted the machine to what I thought was a reasonable level and flipped the switch. Michelle yelled out, turned blue ...

... and stopped breathing.

We resuscitated her. But she spent the next three days under observation in the Pediatric ICU and some of the staff there were furious with me. There is a certain amount of rivalry among physicians and our missteps tend to be remembered. Almost immediately, people started calling me Shock Doc. I'd get asked if I had zapped anyone lately. I still hear about it from time to time, even after all these years.

It wasn't one of my career highlights. It was definitely not the result I had been looking for.

As far as I was concerned, that was the end of the experiment. Never again would I attempt Russian stimulation on a young child. But if I was ready to give up on the idea, her parents weren't and neither were some of the nurses. They took to buttonholing me every chance they got. And because Michelle's ward was between my office and the NICU, they had plenty of opportunity to corner me. I could be called in during the middle of the night and walking down the hall at two o'clock in the morning and one of the nurses would come out of the nurses' station and start arguing with me. They understood that the first attempt to use electrical stimulation had gone wrong, but they were convinced the theory of muscle weakness was valid. They wanted me to figure out some way to help her. They were relentless, well-meaning nags.

Eventually they wore me down.

Obviously, I wasn't going to repeat the disaster of the first experiment, but after thinking about it, I wondered if there might be a way to achieve a better result by making a simple adjustment to the technology. Russian stimulation is high-intensity stimulation applied for a short period. (They keep it short because, even for adults, it's uncomfortable.) This being the case, I reasoned, why not try low-intensity stimulation for a longer period?

I had to go back to the ethics panel. They said okay—just don't make her stop breathing.

Michelle didn't like me by now. I couldn't get near her without her acting up. She was definitely not going to take kindly to having electrodes attached to her body again, so we had to resort to subterfuge. We did it at night, when she was asleep. And this seemed to work: she slept peacefully while the machine quietly sent low-level electrical pulses through her torso. I had a research fellow who lived in the residence across the road and he volunteered to help out. He would come in after dinner, set up the machine, and leave it to the nurses to detach the electrodes in the morning. We repeated this routine night after night for a few weeks.

The results were astonishing.

One day, after about five weeks of electrical stimulation, Michelle was on the mat and she pushed herself up into the sitting position and said, "Look! Look at me! Look what I've done!"

And then she just took off.

Within six months she was able to crawl, control her bladder, and be taken off the ventilator for longer periods of time. After eight months she was up and walking in a walker. She still needed the ventilator to breathe for her when she was asleep, but over the years that followed, she got to the point that when she was awake she could breathe on her own, without assistance.

Two years later, at age seven, Michelle moved to the old Bloorview Children's Hospital. She required full-time observation as she needed frequent suctioning and was connected to the ventilator at night during sleep. She was there until she was fourteen, attending school and having short home visits. When she started high school, she moved home.

— • —

Therapeutic electrical stimulation (TES), the name I initially gave to the nighttime version of NMES, had proven itself in its first tryout. It had worked for Michelle, but was it a fluke? Was something else going on in Michelle's case that I had failed to take into account? You can't base a new therapeutic strategy on a single success. I wanted to try it out on my patients with cerebral palsy. We knew that the muscles in CP are also weak due to limited activity and the side effect of braces. Would TES work with them as well?

I set up a pilot study with cooperation from the Hospital for Sick Children and financial support from the Ontario Easter Seals Research Institute.[3] I looked for ex-premature children who had been diagnosed with mild spastic diplegia or hemiplegia. I especially wanted to test the technique on children whose disability was mild—contrary to the usual practice of trying out a new therapy on the most severely affected patients.[4]

Two boys and three girls in the Toronto area took part in the study, all between three and six years of age, with mild spastic hemiplegia or diplegia. They were all able to walk independently. They were bright children with no suggestion of an intellectual deficit, just a physical impairment. All of them continued in their regular therapy programs in the community.

We started with a baseline test using the Peabody Developmental Motor Scales (PDMS), which is used to assess gross and fine motor function. We made sure that the people doing the testing had no knowledge of the research protocol. There were also three control children: one was a twin to a study subject and the other two were triplet siblings of another. They had the same baseline testing as their siblings. The parents were given a TES unit—it was about the size of a paperback book—and the electrodes that went with it, plus instructions on how to fix the pads onto the child's body. We left it up to them to decide whether to turn the machine on before or after the child went to sleep. We gave them a diary so they could keep track of sleep times and any functional changes, and to let us know if they missed any nights of stimulation. And we checked up on them periodically, to make sure the electrodes were being positioned correctly and the machines were working. We had them use the machines for six nights a week for six months and then told them to stop.

The children would be on TES for six months, off for six months, on TES again for six months, and finally off again for six months. At the end of each half-year stretch they would be tested again with the PDMS, which tests a wide range of motor skills, and have a neurologic assessment. The idea was to see whether they would improve more during the six-month periods of therapy than during the six months when they were off of it.

We did the same with the children who were included in the study as control subjects.

At the end of the study, we found that during the periods of TES treatment, children improved far more than they did during the off periods. The one area measured by the Peabody tests where nothing much happened was in non-locomotor skills, such as stretching, bending, and twisting. In other words, TES did not make the children more supple; it served only to increase motor function. As for the control children, they showed no significant change beyond age-appropriate increases in function.

Even though very few children were included in this study, this was an *extremely* significant result. The statistical probability of this happening by chance was one in a thousand. It clearly showed that TES had a beneficial effect for children with mild-severity cerebral palsy.

All the children with CP who completed the study showed positive change. The mildest cases showed the most improvement, which is hardly surprising, but all the children improved. When looked at again two years later, some were still using TES, and still getting better. Rehabilitation therapy remained essential, but TES seemed to be a powerful addition to the therapists' inventory of tools.

— • —

When I first tried low-level TES with Michelle, I assumed the electrical impulse stimulated muscle growth directly, but I later came to realize that this was not the case. The voltage was so low that it wasn't actually causing the muscles to contract, which is what happened when NMES was used. Because the muscle was not contracting, originally there was some resistance from therapists to using TES. It was hard to understand what was happening when the current was giving just a sensory-level stimulation. At best, we were stimulating blood flow. Years after the publication of our first pilot study, I changed the name of the technique from therapeutic electrical stimulation to threshold electrical stimulation. The stimulation level that I had stumbled into using with Michelle was just at the sensory threshold, barely perceptible and definitely different from the jolting stimulation of NMES. Also, just to confuse the matter, the name therapeutic electrical stimulation in Europe is used to describe what we in North America call NMES.

But TES did change the weak muscles and we could see and feel the change in about six to eight weeks. A weak muscle looks smaller than normal and is soft and almost spongy to the touch, like an uncooked chicken breast. Parents reported that in the first two months of use, the muscle started to look bigger, but it still was weaker than normal. When gently prodded or massaged, it started to feel like partially cooked chicken breast. Another observation was that as the repetitive sensory stimulation of TES was transmitted to the brain, the child gradually became more aware of the muscle and started to use it. I did not understand fully what was going on at this stage, but later, when I taught therapists how to use TES, I told them to watch for growth first and when they could see and feel change in the treated muscles, start to actively strengthen them.

There was another feature of Michelle's case that I did not understand until several years later. Both an adult and an infant get weaker in the aftermath of a spinal cord injury. They're in hospital, they're in spinal shock, and they're unable to move. The difference between them is that the adult knows he's weak. He understands the problem and works to get stronger. The infant doesn't know. She has no memory of having moved her hands or of standing and walking. She's handicapped not only by weakness but also by inexperience, and both the weakness and the sheer novelty of movement have to be dealt with in the course of rehabilitation. There are two challenges to be met, not just one.

Michelle illustrated both issues—weakness and inexperience—perfectly because her brain was spared the damage that affected her spinal cord: it was plain to see that her inability to move was secondary to the spinal cord injury. Knowing that it was a secondary effect made all the difference. Once we realized that her nerves were recovered enough to transmit brain signals to produce the weak movements, it meant that her motor impairment could be treated.

—— • ——

While I still was at HSC, I initiated another research project, this one supported by the Ontario March of Dimes, to gauge the effectiveness of TES in adults with post-polio syndrome.

In the 1950s, there had been two major epidemics in North America of poliomyelitis, a vicious disease that causes partial paralysis and in some cases death. It has now been virtually eradicated by a comprehensive program of vaccination. Many of those who survived the initial bout with polio were left with some level of disability.

In the late 1980s, at the time I was experimenting with TES, post-polio syndrome was disrupting the lives of something like 50 percent of polio survivors as they approached middle age. Many had symptoms that matched those of adults with cerebral palsy: increasing weakness in the muscles that had been attacked by the initial problem, chronic fatigue, and problems with balance. In effect, they had muscle weakness without any of the traits that complicated experiments with children. They weren't subject to growth spurts. Their brains and personalities were fully developed. The incidence of spontaneous recovery was nil. I thought that by working with post-polio survivors I could measure the effects of low-level electrical stimulation on muscle growth and strength while controlling for factors that might complicate the results of trials with children.

I also had a new tool to measure outcomes. Professor Michael Joy, who was the associate director of biomedical engineering at U of T, had access to an experimental magnetic resonance imaging (MRI) unit. He became a co-principal investigator of the research study in charge of using the MRI to measure muscle mass in patients with post-polio syndrome treated by TES: with his assistance we could tell definitively if muscles were growing or gaining in size.

The Ontario March of Dimes put out a call for people who had been hit by post-polio syndrome. The trial was up and running when I met Catherine Bell, an accomplished woman whose solid and fulfilling career had been upset by the onset of post-polio syndrome.

— • —

Catherine was two years old when she was struck by polio. It was 1953. "I woke up screaming and holding my legs," she says. Their family doctor diagnosed it as polio and Catherine was taken to the Hospital for Sick Children in Toronto. She stayed there for two weeks before being transferred to a convalescent hospital in another part of the city, and there she remained in quarantine for about two months. All that time, her parents scarcely saw her: they were allowed to visit only once a month. This was standard practice for hospitalized children in those days. She has no memory of the stay, but her father recalled that all the parents came to visit at the same time and when they left the wailing and crying of the children filled the halls. He said that no one should have to hear that.

It was mainly the nerves controlling her lower limbs and abdomen that were affected by the poliovirus. Catherine was operated on when she was two years old, again at four, when she was eleven, and then again when she was sixteen and seventeen. "At age seventeen I was able to walk normally. No one knew I had polio unless I was tired. I could wear high heels. I could skate. I could run."

Catherine studied fashion design, and when she applied for a job with a knitwear manufacturer, she mentioned her medical history. The manager said the job involved travel. He said she would have to carry her own suitcase and cope with train stations and a lot of walking, and he wanted to know if she would have a problem with that. She said no, she had put polio behind her, and she was as good as her word. "He was a workaholic who walked very quickly, six foot four and I'm only five foot three, and I kept up with him for fourteen years."

She was in her mid-thirties when things started to go wrong.

"I'd fall and my husband would be looking for me in the kitchen and I would be on the floor. My left quad became quite weak and the knee would give way." She took a bad fall down a flight of stairs, tearing some ligaments and ending up in a cast. They were living in a house with a lot of stairs and her husband had stair glides installed. And she found herself tiring easily. She started using a scooter to get around the factory. She catnapped in the afternoon in her office. She started using a cane. Ultimately, it became too much. She resigned and took a job teaching at a community college.

She got in touch with the March of Dimes to find out what might be done about her deteriorating physical condition. Through them, she started attending support-group meetings in Toronto. It was at one of these meetings that she heard me give a talk about my research. She approached me and I agreed to include her in this trial. This was in 1989.

Before she heard me speak, she said, no one had given her any reason to think that she could recover. If anything, the therapists she encountered were discouraging. "They said stop overdoing your exercises. You can get in the water and do non-fatiguing exercises, have naps and so on." They were telling her to conserve her strength rather than rebuild it.

We ran a baseline MRI on Catherine's leg and gave her a TES machine to take home with her. "We first worked on just the quadriceps muscle for eleven months," said Catherine. "Six nights a week, I would put two electrodes on my leg above the knee and at the top of the thigh and go to bed with it." Within weeks she noticed changes: better balance, improved circulation, and discernible growth in the wasted thigh muscles.

The second MRI was done at eleven months. The *before* picture showed the muscle marbled with fat with small pockets of normal-looking muscle. The *after* picture had very little marbling. The overall size of her muscles did not change much, but there were definite changes in the ratio of muscle to fat.

After the trial, Catherine continued to use the TES machine independently. She was also using a Wet Vest to do deep-water jogging. Overall, the combination of TES and non-fatiguing exercise had made a huge difference in her life. She donated her scooter to the March of Dimes. For several years she even dispensed with the cane. Twenty-five years have gone by and Catherine has another business now. She's an image consultant running seminars for corporate clients. She carries a cane but it's mainly for balance. And she's absolutely convinced that TES made the difference in turning her life around.

seven

Personalized Neurorehabilitation

The small studies I had done at the Hospital for Sick Children demonstrated that TES had a positive effect on weak muscles. It was an exciting start, and the results that I saw in my patients were so positive that I started to shift my focus from the diagnosis and prevention of brain injury in the NICU to investigating what else could be done to help children with cerebral palsy.

I was much younger then, and I was optimistic that I could make the switch inside the walls of Sick Kids, the hospital that had been so good to me in my career. By then, I had developed some considerable clout inside the hospital. My colleagues had elected me president of the medical staff. I served on the hospital's board and ethics committee, several key search committees, and the new hospital building committee and contributed to the design of the new NICU.

As an associate professor of pediatrics, I did research studies and had cross appointments at the University of Toronto's Institute of Biomedical Engineering, the Department of Community Health (Division of Exercise Sciences), and the School of Graduate Studies.

Initially I tried to open a new clinic at Sick Kids with the dual aim of developing new therapies for young patients and running research trials to determine their efficacy. Yet I ran into opposition from the administration, from the neurologists, and particularly from the new head of the Neonatal ICU, who had no interest in what I was doing. His focus was firmly within the confines of neonatal research and clinical care. The best that he would offer me was the use of a limited clinic space for three hours on Friday afternoons.

The atmosphere was becoming strained for other reasons as well. The hospital Research Institute was making a deliberate effort to shift research support towards molecular and genetic research. The type of clinical research that I wanted to do had fallen out of favour. As a result, a large number of physicians and surgeons, many of them first-rate clinicians and teachers, were being quietly forced out and replaced with physician-scientists. There is politics in medicine, just as there is in any profession, and a new regime was taking over.

I eventually understood that if I wanted to help children with brain damage get better, as Michelle had done, I couldn't do it inside the hospital. I left the Hospital for Sick Children to open the Magee Clinic at the end of 1989. By early 1991, I was working with two pediatricians, a physiatrist, a massage therapist, and a NICU nurse who had worked with me at the Follow-Up Clinic at HSC. I also had a series of part-time therapists and co-op students from the kinesiology programs at the Universities of Guelph and Waterloo.

The clinic was designed as an open observational trial of new approaches to the assessment and treatment of early-acquired neurologic problems. This meant that everyone, including our patients and the staff, knew precisely what was happening and everything was assessed. Two members of the Hospital for Sick Children's ethics board agreed to sit on the clinic's ethics committee, as well as a lawyer who had an interest in the subject, and a couple of parents whose children we were treating. When a child was referred to the clinic from a distance, we sent out a video documentation request with instructions on how to make a tape of the child's performance on a standardized series of activities that assessed upper- and lower-limb abilities. A clinic physician reviewed this tape, along with the medical history, before an appointment was made. Inappropriate candidates, ones we thought we would be unable to help, were refused at this stage. I set up a protocol for each clinic visit that included standardized testing of function, again documented on videotape, as well as a therapy assessment and EMG biofeedback test (more on this below), plus a neurologic examination by one of the clinic physicians on every patient visit. During this time, we created a new technique to document trunk weakness[1] and established the reliability of using videotaped assessments of standardized tests.[2]

In addition to the clinic work, I had an active lecture schedule, giving lectures and grand rounds in hospitals and clinics throughout the United States and Canada on my new approach, challenging the old theory that the best we could hope for in children with cerebral palsy was "some improvement in their limitations."[3] On these trips, I made it a routine to ask to speak with therapists as well as the physicians and surgeons and, whenever possible, joined the therapists as an observer in their sessions to actually watch children being treated. I was surprised to find that there were many different treatment techniques and technologies in common use. On trips overseas, I learned of other approaches. Children were getting treatment everywhere, but what was available to the individual child at any particular centre seemed to be limited to the training and preference of the therapist.

My approach developed over time into what would now be called personalized medical care, as offered in executive health programs and specialized diagnostic centres throughout North America. This is common today, but in the 1990s, it was a new and unfamiliar approach. The mission of all the clinic staff was to first assess each patient's weaknesses, but also his strengths, and then come up with a comprehensive and customized treatment plan that included recommending interventions from all the professional silos involved in the care of the patient. At the time, this type of comprehensive diagnostic assessment and forward planning was not a routine part of the ongoing treatment of patients with stable, chronic neurologic problems. Back then, the common wisdom was to prevent an expected deterioration and not give parents *false hope* of achieving significant improvement.

Our goal was to provide a fresh look at the whole patient and to design a personalized one-year plan for improvement with measurable metrics to document any change. The patient population included children of all ages with a wide variety of diagnoses. The common thread was brain, spinal cord, or nerve damage. Their conditions were all considered stable and chronic, with an established expectation of limited change.

I was happy to assess them all, just as I was happy to explore different options in the treatment of post-polio syndrome. It was as much about problem solving as it was about medicine. It was about developing approaches that worked, such as TES, which helped at least some patients improve. The majority of patients were children or adults with cerebral palsy, but there were also children with spina bifida (an abnormality of development of the lower spinal cord) and brachial plexus injury (or BPI, a birth injury to the nerves controlling movement of one arm). When one of the rehabilitation specialists (a physiatrist) from the local spinal cord injury rehabilitation hospital joined the staff, we also saw adults with late-stage spinal cord injuries, most of whom were thought to be beyond the possibility of further recovery. Another part-time adult physiatrist brought patients with stroke and chronic pain syndromes. I was appointed for a short time at Lyndhurst, a Toronto spinal cord injury rehabilitation hospital, where we wrote grants and tried to initiate a pilot trial of TES in patients with more acute spinal cord injury. Unfortunately, the program was not funded.

This is another common problem in academic research. As Kuhn pointed out in 1962, the practitioners of normal science have the power and prestige to preside over grant review boards where, not surprisingly, they tend to actively resist new ideas. Young investigators, or those new to a field, have a notoriously difficult time breaking the barriers to stable funding, particularly for studies labelled clinical research.[4] I was frustrated by this resistance, but consoled myself with the knowledge that I was in good company.

At the Magee Clinic, we were deliberately eclectic in our practice. I had made a break from the hospital setting, where diagnosis and research had been my overwhelming preoccupation, to explore therapies that offered the promise of changing outcomes for patients whose progress I previously had mostly just monitored. Michelle had precipitated a profound change in my outlook. I had caught a glimpse of what might be possible and the point now was to do something about it. We did not at any time promise miracle cures. Some cases (roughly 20 to 30 percent of patients referred by their physicians to the clinic) we gently turned away because we couldn't give them a real chance to improve. For the patients that we thought could improve, we would use TES if we thought it would help. For each patient, we tried to match, as best we could, the available treatments and technologies to the needs of the patient and the family. We worked with physical and occupational therapists and, for a short while, a speech therapist.

When it was appropriate, we referred patients to specialists, including neurosurgeons and orthopedic surgeons. An operation to treat spasticity, selective dorsal rhizotomy (SDR), was increasingly available in the United States, as were a growing range of innovative orthopedic surgeries. We recommended other new treatments, like Botox and intrathecal

Baclofen pumps. The pumps were in widespread use for adult spinal cord injury and were now being offered in a few specialized centres to children as well. Whatever worked we were willing to study and, if appropriate, offer to our patients. In every case, our job was the overall assessment and creation of a one-year plan of action. This was communicated to both the family and the referring physician and therapists, who supervised the program locally. Unfortunately, many of the newer treatments were not yet available in Canada. I did not think it was my job to withhold information about new research findings, and we willingly arranged referrals to recognized centres. As experience with this more active intervention model grew, so did the number of repeat referrals and invitations to lecture, particularly in the United States.

— • —

Fairly early into the Magee Clinic years, I realized that many of the training principles I had been taught by a great series of tennis coaches could be applied to children with cerebral palsy. When I was young, I remember a coach at a junior tennis intensive camp told us that as girls, we had about 40 percent less upper-body muscle mass than boys of the same size. Too bad, he told us, it's genetics. He claimed weakness was a significant factor in sports-related injuries and that these injuries were more common in girls. So, he added bilateral upper-body and trunk strengthening programs to our regular drills. I think he was the first to point out to me that puberty was a significant opportunity for growth. At the clinic, I put this sports wisdom together with the realization that many of the preteens and teens that used crutches to walk were coming to the clinic complaining of increasing shoulder pain as they grew and gained weight. It seemed obvious that they could benefit from more shoulder strength as they grew through puberty.

I did not realize at first that prescribing active resistance exercises to teens with cerebral palsy was a challenge to another of those "common wisdom" beliefs in the therapy world. At the time, therapists in North America were taught that strength training in children with spasticity was wrong and that strengthening might actually make a child with CP worse. Yet, in travels to Scandinavia, I visited adapted circuit-training programs for teenagers to do after-school group strength training. This type of differing belief system was a recurring event. In North America, we are indebted to Diane Damiano and her colleagues at the National Institutes of Health for dismantling this incorrect idea.[5] Both strength training, properly done, and intensive active training protocols are now accepted as good therapy interventions for children with CP.[6]

Indeed, it was obvious that whatever mechanism of strengthening we employed, a choice in part determined by individual and family preference, a program of strengthening enhanced the result. I was also discovering the remarkable therapeutic possibilities of water and developed a water exercise program using the Wet Vest, a neutral buoyancy device that allowed children and adults to walk and jog in deep water, with their heads held out of the water. A competitive runner first developed this technique to help him recover after a war injury. It is now widely used in the rehabilitation of professional athletes and U.S. military personnel. For the child or adult with a neurologic problem, it was an inexpensive, effective way of providing access to out-of-gravity exercise. Learning how to stay upright and then move about a pool was a novel challenge that rapidly took the child "out of habit" and revealed underlying recovery. It was not unusual to have a child who walked with difficulty learn to jog in the water within minutes, moving all four limbs in a reciprocal pattern.

— • —

While the clinic was in operation, we saw five hundred to one thousand new patients a year. We got a lot of positive media in newspapers and magazines and on television. CNN sent a crew to Toronto to interview Michelle, her mother, and me. By this time Michelle was walking well in a walker and attending school at Bloorview. She came to the clinic for the day to be interviewed and she was the star of the show. As it turned out, the piece was one of the news network's best-received health reports. It was replayed for years on CNN International, attracting inquiries and patients from surprisingly distant locations. If we proved nothing else, we showed that there was a hunger out there for a positive, new approach to the old problem of cerebral palsy and other early neurologic problems.

A contributor to a newsletter for the Ontario Spina Bifida Association described what a patient could expect on a visit to the clinic in its early days:

The initial assessment was conducted over two or three days.... Videos were made to record the child's range of abilities and realistic goals were set. No miracles were promised. A youth in a wheelchair was not led to believe that he would soon be running, but standing was held out as a distinct possibility. Nothing, however, would come without work. The treatment was presented, not as an overnight project, but rather as one that might take months or years.[7]

— • —

I was open to adopting any device or treatment that offered hope for making a positive change in the lives of our patients. As I have mentioned, I tried to keep up with how researchers in the wider neuroscience world were using innovative techniques to stimulate brain neuroplasticity. I presented our pilot results using TES in patients with chronic spinal cord injury at a meeting of the Spinal Cord Society in the United States. At that meeting, I heard about the use of surface electromyographic (EMG) biofeedback at the University of Miami. Some of the patients I saw in Toronto had been there for an intensive period of training and they were happy with the results.

I went for a two-week training program with Bernie Brucker at the Spinal Cord Injury Unit at the University of Miami. Bernie was an inspiring clinician and innovator. He was committed to finding ways to help restore function to people with disabilities—and one of the tools he used was EMG biofeedback. It was in Miami that I first saw a multi-lead surface EMG unit make magic in minutes. I watched him work with adults recovering from a spinal cord injury and teenagers with cerebral palsy. All of them had trouble moving their limbs normally. Bernie attached stick-on electrodes to the target muscles and the machine then recorded small baseline signals from the muscles on a monitor. Then came the magic. He would ask the patients to "think about" moving their foot or arm while watching the computer screen. As they thought about moving the limb, the baseline EMG signal would move! Then he asked them to make the line move up and down and they quickly learned how to take control and move the limb. The little EMG signals, translated to a moving line on a screen, gave them accurate feedback of the movements of their muscles. And as Bernie said, "It is all about feedback. If you see it change, you can make it change." I started to use it too.

We used EMG biofeedback to help older children and adults with cerebral palsy learn how to decrease their spastic tone. We would attach electrodes over both the spastic and non-spastic muscles in pairs so that the machine recorded and displayed muscle activity on a computer screen. This gave the patient a visual representation of what was happening when the tight or spastic muscle overpowered its weaker antagonist. Given this real-time feedback, the patient learned first to turn off the overactive spastic muscle and then to activate, and over time strengthen, the antagonist with specific, practised movements. Although there was little in the way of research to justify its use at that time, we found it to be an effective tool for treating upper-limb dysfunction and in gait training. Because some cognitive skill and discipline are needed, it was less effective in treating very young children. Nevertheless, we found that children as young as five years could be taught to use their personal "video game."

— • —

Lisa was about six or seven when I met her. She had moderate spastic diplegia, a type of cerebral palsy that affected only her legs. She would be classified as a Level III on the GMFCS. She could stand briefly and walked independently with bilateral forearm crutches and bilateral ankle foot orthoses (AFOs). These are the most commonly used braces to assist walking in children with CP. She found it difficult to lift up (dorsiflex) her foot at the ankle. When she tried, the tightness or excess tone in the muscles at the back of her leg would pull her toes down and her ankle up, the exact opposite of what we wanted her to do. No matter how hard she tried, the spastic muscles would fire first and overpower the weaker muscles on the front of her leg.

So Andy, our kinesiology co-op student, hooked her up with electrodes on the front and back of the leg while she sat in front of the computer monitor. He showed her the signal on the screen that recorded movement of the spastic muscles on the back of her leg and asked her to make the line go down. It took her only a few minutes to learn how to lower the line by voluntarily relaxing the tight muscles. Then he moved the electrodes to the non-spastic antagonist muscles on the front of her leg and, even though the signal was weak, he was able to teach her how to lift the line up and then lower it. All this time, she had her eyes on the screen: she seemed not to be aware that her foot was now moving up and down; the line on the screen claimed all her attention. After a few minutes, we asked her to look at her foot. Her mouth dropped open and she said, "That's what dorsiflexion is!" For years her parents and therapists had encouraged her to dorsiflex her foot, but she couldn't do it. She knew the word and what she was supposed to do, but until she actually saw and felt her foot moving upwards, she really didn't "know" it. Less than thirty minutes with accurate biofeedback from her muscles changed all that. It was an aha! moment and a significant milestone in her treatment.

I made an EMG biofeedback session standard for all new patients, in part to help us understand the extent of their problem, but also to create moments like these. Once the patients—and families—could see their underlying ability, it was easier to motivate them to do the hard work to improve function.

This was all new in the early 1990s, but pioneering doctors at major institutions like Harvard University were starting to use different types of biofeedback and mindfulness training to help people reduce stress and lower their blood pressure. This is now accepted standard practice and a useful part of the cardiologist's toolbox. The approach was thought to be radical at the time, but gradually it became conventional wisdom that if the brain receives accurate information from the senses, it is able to learn and change. In the 1990s, this new idea was starting to creep into the world of adult treatment, but little of this knowledge was influencing the world of pediatric neurorehabilitation at that time.

——— • ———

Patients came to us from all over the world. They had to be referred to us by their doctors and sometimes getting a referral wasn't easy. Norah Myers was born prematurely at St. Boniface Hospital in Winnipeg in 1984. She suffered two brain hemorrhages shortly after birth. As her mother, Barbara, related, "They told us they didn't know what effect the hemorrhages would have. We could only wait and see."

Norah started therapy early and as she grew, her parents continued to work with her. She had a minor visual impairment that she learned to work around, but her main problem was muscle weakness, more obvious on the left than on the right side. "She learned to walk," said Barbara. "She had an in-shoe orthotic similar to ones used by athletes and runners everywhere to correct foot malalignment. She fell sometimes, but she was independent. She was still stumbling in kindergarten, but she held her own."

It was obvious from the start that Norah was smart. She attended an elementary public school and did well, although her minor disability tended to set her apart socially. It bothered her parents that the problem appeared to be permanent. Even with exercise and therapy, her weakness didn't go away.

Barbara heard about the Magee Clinic when Norah was seven. A therapist, Kim Schmidt, now Barthel, told her about it. Barbara got in touch, and I sent her a cassette tape recording of a conference where I'd been a speaker. When Barbara said she wanted me to see Norah, I told her to ask her pediatrician for a referral. He wouldn't give it to her. He said that the clinic's work wasn't published and he wasn't convinced that the therapy worked.

Barbara called another doctor and got a similar response. She worked her way through the Winnipeg phone book. "I called every pediatrician I could get a hold of, at least a dozen. I called them all. They all said the same thing. They refused to give me a referral. Finally I found one. He saw Norah, examined her, and wrote the letter for me.

"We had liftoff."

— • —

The resistance Barbara Myers encountered when she sought assistance from her doctor wasn't unusual. The approach we were offering at the Magee Clinic was new and some doctors were suspicious. We were getting a good deal of publicity in popular media, and while that exposure attracted patients, it probably repelled some physicians. Like many professionals, they doubt the capacity of ordinary reporters to assess medical innovations accurately. We were careful to emphasize to every reporter who came to visit us that we were not claiming to make miracles happen. We stressed the long-term commitment that was required of patients. We made it clear that the various treatment recommendations and technologies we were employing were varied to suit each patient's unique situation. Everyone was different. We did what we could to anticipate and respond to criticism. We were criticized just the same.

In January 1993, the *Canadian Medical Association Journal* published an article written by a freelance writer, Olga Lechky, that gave a positive account of our work. While much of the article focused on our use of TES and EMG feedback, the writer picked up on the underlying argument about neuroplasticity. "By wedding the laboratory concept of neuroplasticity—the apparent ability of the brain either to repair damaged areas over time or to find alternate pathways around an injury—to new home-based technologies that stimulate repair mechanisms," she wrote, "Pape and her colleagues have offered new hope to more than 2,000 patients since the Magee Clinic opened its doors in 1989."[8]

This made a number of doctors very unhappy and they expressed their displeasure in letters to the CMA journal.[9]

James G. Wright, an orthopedic surgeon based at my old stomping ground at the Hospital for Sick Children in Toronto, declared his belief "that the article provides an unbalanced view of the benefits of electrical stimulation and could give unreasonable hope of cure to a vulnerable group of children and their families."

"I hope that Pape's desire to pursue clinical trials is realized," wrote Robert W. Teasell, M.D., from London, Ontario. "Until then, clinicians should maintain a healthy degree of scepticism before recommending TES to patients with chronic neurologic impairment, many of whom are vulnerable and eager to grasp at any potential treatment."

Peter Rosenbaum, M.D., and his colleagues in Hamilton, Ontario, complained about the lack of peer-reviewed scientific articles to justify the use of the clinic's treatments. He wondered "if this is because the group does not see the importance of sharing their findings with their peers (an odd situation considering Dr. Pape's output in her previous career as a neonatologist) or whether the results do not meet peer-reviewed standards of scientific merit and credibility."

Finally, Robert Armstrong, M.D., from Vancouver, British Columbia, wrote, "I know of no published evidence, other than in abstracts and articles in non-peer-reviewed journals, of the effectiveness of the treatment for the populations described in the article." He took his complaint one step further, writing, "Publishing articles like this does harm and compromises the credibility of the healthcare system."

Perhaps, given this outpouring, it was not surprising that some physicians across the land were reluctant to refer their patients to the Magee Clinic.

In response to the critics, the journal's editors defended their decision to publish Lechky's article. They pointed out that it was printed as news, not as a scientific review or endorsement. And as news, they wrote, "The popularity of the clinic alone justifies publication." They concluded their editorial, "Regardless of whether TES has real therapeutic value, patients continue to go to the clinic because it offers something that they have not received from other healthcare services. We believe that the Lechky article will stimulate physicians to think about what TES really offers and will stimulate believers in TES to prove its worth or otherwise."[10]

The editors also gave me the opportunity to respond to the critics. In my letter I pointed out that the clinic had prepared eleven abstracts, "all of which were peer-reviewed before their presentation to the Canadian Paediatric Society, the Society for Pediatric Research, the American Academy for Cerebral Palsy and Developmental Medicine, the Canadian Congress of Neurological Sciences and the American Academy of Pediatrics." I observed that even some of the critics had acknowledged improvement in their patients.

"This debate is really about testing new ideas," I wrote. "Initially a researcher must be convinced that a study is warranted. Then the study must be designed, funded, completed, analysed, reported and published. The delay can be as long as 5 or 10 years."[11] And once this last stage is completed, then others repeat the study to see if the findings are reproducible. In other words, I pointed out that my detractors appeared to be demanding proof of an experiment whose outlines had not yet been fully explored or designed.

Part of my irritation with them was that they seemed to be demanding a different standard for new techniques than what they were currently offering as common practice in their treatment clinics. It is a well-recognized fact in all areas of medicine that many of the tried-and-true treatments in common, accepted usage have never been subjected to rigorous research trials. It takes time to gain acceptance for new ideas.

An article I wrote with colleagues for the journal *Contemporary Pediatrics* gives an accurate indication of my thinking at around this time. I wrote, "At least three different processes contribute to the final disability: first is the primary lesion to the nervous system, affecting the child's 'control' system; the second is a disturbance of muscle and bone growth; and the third is a learned response, as the child develops abnormal movement patterns to compensate for the neural damage."[12] The child in this condition, having no concept of normal movement, learns to move abnormally. In designing a treatment plan for improvement, each component—the brain damage, the spasticity and body distortion, and the maladaptive habits—needs attention and a very different therapeutic approach.

— • —

What about my critics' complaint that more research was needed? When I was still at Sick Kids, the ethics committee decided, in effect, that I could not ethically run a randomized controlled trial to test the effects of threshold electrical stimulation. They argued that it would be unethical for me to withhold treatment from a control group because I would be withholding a therapy that I believed was effective. The essence of an RCT is the assumption that the researcher is unbiased: she doesn't know if it will work or not. The committee members said it was obvious that I was biased because I "knew" TES worked. They suggested that I have other researchers undertake the trials.

Over the next few years, I worked with several groups that expressed interest in doing a randomized controlled trial of TES. This type of trial is considered the gold standard when it comes to medical research. The idea is that subjects, rather than being cherry-picked because they're likely to respond positively to treatment, are chosen at random. The experiment is "controlled" by having a second group of subjects who match the description of the first group, but from whom treatment is withheld, the idea being to make sure that whatever happens to the first group isn't a spontaneous development but a direct response to the treatment. There are other rules and conventions to minimize the chance of experimenter or other biases, but the most important component of the RCT is to make sure that the comparison groups are equivalent. Unfortunately, in children with cerebral palsy, there are a very large number of interacting variables and failure to adequately control these has led to great difficulty in neurorehabilitation research. The reason our first TES trial produced extremely significant results with a small study sample is that we had controlled possible confounding variables extremely well. All the subjects were born prematurely and were between three and six years of age at the time of the study. They had normal intelligence, vision, and hearing. Their only problem was mild-severity cerebral palsy.

In the pediatric neurorehabilitation literature it is not uncommon to see study samples with a wide range of age and severity and a modest sample size. This practice offends the principles of good research design and what we know about developmental neuroplasticity. Every parent knows that the brain of a five-year-old child is not comparable with that of a fifteen-year-old teenager.

Only one positive randomized controlled trial of TES has been conducted. Dr. Paul Steinbok and physiotherapist

Ann Reiner at the University of British Columbia designed a well-controlled study that produced clear proof of positive change.[13] The study patients were children with the spastic diplegic form of cerebral palsy who had undergone selective dorsal rhizotomy at least a year earlier. An SDR is a neurosurgical procedure in which the neurosurgeon cuts a proportion of the sensory nerve fibres from the spastic muscles in the leg at the level of the spinal cord. This reduces the abnormal increased tone in the legs. Spastic muscles are already weak; the surgical denervation (cutting the sensory nerves) weakens the muscle even more. The research question was whether or not TES could act effectively to redress the balance.

The patients were very similar, ranging in age from four to ten years old, averaging about seven. They were a homogeneous group of children with cerebral palsy who had all previously qualified for the SDR surgery. One group was given TES and a second group wasn't. Regular therapy interventions were continued for both groups. The children who were treated with TES used the unit for eight to twelve hours a night, a minimum of six nights a week, for twelve months. They were given a baseline assessment using the Gross Motor Function Measure (GMFM), which was then repeated at six months and on completion of the trial at twelve months by trained evaluators with no knowledge (blinded) of the treatment status of the patients. The outcome was positive: "The results," wrote Steinbok, "indicated a statistically significant improvement in outcome for the treated children using the GMFM, with the difference in means between the two groups being 3.6%. The extent of improvement is considered to be clinically important ... and is reflected in the greater functional gains in the treated, compared with non-treated, children.... This was in keeping with the observations of the primary caregivers with respect to the changes they noted in the treated versus untreated children."[14]

The language is academic and restrained, but this was a well-designed, positive RCT. Yet, in spite of this result, no one has repeated the trial with a wider group of children post-rhizotomy, nor is TES widely recommended or used for the post-operative rehabilitation of children after an SDR. Part of the problem in disseminating the results of this trial may have been that the paper was published in a pediatric neurorehabilitation journal not regularly read by other neurosurgeons. As I have discussed in Chapter 5, specialized knowledge in healthcare is often limited to each professional silo. Even within a hospital system there may be such silos. At the same time that Robert Armstrong wrote in to complain about the lack of published research on TES—research that takes time to design, test, and report—this RCT was in progress at his own hospital.

— • —

Meanwhile, some of the neurologists at the Hospital for Sick Children remained convinced that I was offering "false hope" to a vulnerable population of patients. They made enough noise that the dean of the medical school at the University of Toronto decided to do an independent review of our procedures and practice. He chose an adult neurologist, who then spent a few days at the clinic. He reviewed a random assortment of charts. He examined patients with me and with other members of the medical staff. He interviewed patients when we weren't present. He also interviewed the occupational therapist, the kinesiologist, the nurse-practitioner, and even members of the administrative staff.

He was amazed to discover that I was doing standardized tests of function on every patient as part of the clinic routine. He reviewed a random selection of clinic charts as well as the entry and follow-up videotapes. He sat in on a few biofeedback sessions and was even more amazed by the results. He could see that the therapies we offered were having tangible, positive results. His letter to the dean was as good as an advertisement for our services and the opposition from the medical community faded away.

But the provincial government didn't. Just when things were settling down, around 1994–95, the Ontario Ministry of Health decided that they were going to "clamp down" on physicians who were treating out-of-province and out-of-country patients. There were a lot of discussions back and forth with people from the ministry: I can't say that they were sympathetic to my cause and I had no way of knowing whom else they might be interviewing. At the same time, I was becoming acutely aware of the disparity between the therapy support that was being offered to patients from the United States and those from Canada. The fact was that the children from the States who were able to travel to Canada to see me were routinely given more ongoing therapy back home than was available to most Canadians and their responses to our interventions were more consistent. Judged by the number of repeat referrals, both the therapists and physicians in the United States seemed more open to innovation. The other major factor was that I was getting tired of fighting the Canadian establishment. I decided that my time and skills would be better devoted to introducing therapists and physicians to my model of care, as well as teaching how to use the TES and EMG units, than in soldiering on at the Magee Clinic. Instead of doing it all myself, I would educate others and train them in the techniques so that more patients inside and outside of Canada could benefit from TES and EMG treatment.

I provided the first neuroplasticity and TES workshop to a group of forty therapists in San Francisco in February 1995. In that first year, I taught eleven sessions to over 450 therapists in Canada and the United States. After that year, I closed the Magee Clinic and shifted entirely to an educator mode. I learned a lot personally from my years at the clinic, not least because I started seeing a wider range of patients than I had before. My practice was no longer limited to children with early brain injury. We demonstrated the worth of a number treatments and technologies, used together or in sequence to achieve improvement. We discovered some of the limitations too. Altogether, we made the lives of a large number of patients better. We gave them goals and a plan to follow. We gave them real—not false—hope.

— • —

The first years of the new century brought a number of changes to my life. The Magee Clinic was part of the past. I had started a new company, called the TASC Network, to push forward what I had learned. TASC—Technology-Assisted Self-Care—encapsulated the two concepts I regarded as key to transforming the way children with early neurologic injury are treated. The technology component included TES, as well as EMG biofeedback and EMG-triggered stimulation. It also included a variety of devices to correct dysfunctional alignment caused by spasticity, unbalanced muscle strength, and the movement patterns associated with cerebral palsy. Years earlier, a brilliant physical therapist, Tema Stein, had shown me the difference properly fitted orthotics could make for a child with cerebral palsy who was learning to walk: now the range of splints, braces, and supportive garments available to therapists had increased substantially. Other effective treatments, including Botox, Baclofen pumps, SDR, and innovative orthopedic surgeries, were being offered in major treatment centres. All could be regarded as more or less technological and all held promise for some patients. They were out there but not yet widely used.

The self-care component of the TASC educational program is, perhaps, self-explanatory. More and more, it had become apparent to me that the top-down, physician-as-leader approach to treatment had to be adjusted. Our revolution depended upon parents and patients taking responsibility for their own situation. They knew their child's capabilities better than anyone. They would have to lead the drive to bring about change. It was to them and to the therapists they worked with that I increasingly took my educational message. The revolutions in other areas of healthcare had started with public awareness and patient demand. I reasoned if parents of children knew more about the possibilities inherent in the concept of human neuroplasticity, they would demand more of the neurorehabilitation system in pediatrics. With this is mind, I developed an intensive three- to four-day program for families and therapists; the 20:4:80 program.

The idea implicit in these workshops was that parents are the major decision makers over the first twenty years in the life of a child. I advocated breaking that twenty-year period into sequential four-year plans, like the quadrennial training programs used by Olympic athletes. A talented junior athlete does not train for the Olympics many years in the future. Rather, she trains in four-year intervals, with progressive challenges and different goals for each period. My overall goal was to prepare the child with an early neurologic problem for the normal lifespan that most now achieve. I taught parents that they have the first twenty years to prepare their children for eighty or more years of life as an adult.

My goal was quite simple: Cure for some and improvement for all.

About 80 percent of children with cerebral palsy now have mild to moderate impairment, scoring Level I to III on the most commonly used, standardized scale of function. I had seen some of these children who were effectively cured of their motor disability. I wanted to find out how they managed it. I had seen many more children move from a Level III to a Level II and a Level I to normal. And if they reached this first level of change, their goals could be raised again.

This was the message I set out to take directly to parents in workshops starting in 2000. Many of the parents in attendance knew something about neuroplasticity. Some were aware that, because of it, the standard of care for adult stroke patients had been improved in a big way. But when I told them that the concept had implications for their children, they often looked at me as if I had just landed from outer space. They would ask, "Why wasn't I told?" I took the 20:4:80 program to audiences in the United States, Europe, Israel, South America, and even occasionally back home in Canada. Over the past twenty years I have organized and taught a total of 207 workshops, grand rounds, and lectures to medical and parent groups. I spent a lot of time talking and a lot of time on the road, but after a while, I had to pull back, because family responsibilities with aging parents and changes in my own life required me to prioritize my areas of focus. I held fewer workshops and spent more time reading. I gradually came to the understanding, as I read up on what was happening in adult human neuroscience, that there needed to be a book about the untapped potential of the baby brain. Change was needed and awareness of baby brain neuroplasticity was only the start. I also had discovered that there were ways to improve the function of a child with motor impairments by working with the undamaged parts of the child's brain. Clinical neuroscientists in adult medicine and therapy were discovering untapped resources that also worked in children.

eight

Dance to the Music, Walk with Your Eyes

n 1969, American neuroscientist Paul Bach-y-Rita published a startling letter in *Nature*. He described a "vision substitution machine" that he built to give sight to a person who had been blind from birth.[1] Although he wasn't yet using the term "neuroplasticity," that concept was the premise on which the machine was built. The blind person sat in a large chair with his back pressed against a pad with a mass of embedded electrodes. A camera in front of him sent signals that represented areas of light and shadow in a two-dimensional plane that corresponded to the sheet of electrodes on his back, giving his brain new tactile input to "see" what was in front of him. Amazingly, it worked. The patient, with practice, was able to accurately interpret the signals to identify the shape, position, size, and depth of objects in his field of "vision." He could, in a manner of speaking, see for the first time.

Bach-y-Rita came to refer to what he was doing as "sensory substitution," and he used it to create a range of devices that were meant to use another brain system to retrain the brain. One of his devices was described in Norman Doidge's first book, *The Brain That Changes Itself*.[2] The subject suffered from a rare condition that had robbed her of her vestibular system—the ability to orient herself in space. She couldn't stand, let alone walk. She was described as a "wobbler." Bach-y-Rita's device helped make up for the loss by sending new signals to her brain from a strip of electrodes that sensed movements of her tongue. At first the device worked only while she wore it and for a few seconds after. But the more she wore it, the longer the after-effects lasted, until eventually she completely recovered—or, more precisely, reinvented—her proprioceptive sense. His devices sent novel information to the brain that prompted it to create new neural circuits and acquire new capacities. Later investigators used the tongue as the replacement sensor for sight, allowing a blind climber to climb a mountain using his tongue to sense handholds.[3]

Bach-y-Rita demonstrated that the brain could learn and change how it processes information, substituting different brain systems to restore function.

Activity-dependent neuroplasticity, elegantly demonstrated by Michael Merzenich and his colleagues, showed that the brain uses whatever input it consistently receives. It can learn to recruit other, undamaged parts of the brain to restore lost functions. His book, *Soft-Wired*, covers the wide range of information now available about human neuroplasticity and how we can shape our brains by the information sent to it.[4] But, even in the 1980s and 1990s, we were learning that our brains are a lot more capable than the medical establishment believed.

The following are two stories of using sensory substitution in children with cerebral palsy, training the auditory motor and visuomotor systems to compensate for damage to their motor control system.

Walk to the Music

Sarah was eight years old when I first saw her. It was at a 20:4:80 workshop in Chicago for parents of children with early neurologic damage. Sarah was born early, and as she grew, she developed the classic signs of spastic hemiplegia affecting the function of her left leg, arm, and foot. She walked with a pronounced limp. She had been treated by physiotherapist Pia Stampe, a long-time friend and collaborator of mine. Pia had volunteered to have Sarah demonstrate how music could help her walk better and Sarah came through in a way that surprised us all.

The workshop was held in a large hotel conference room. About 150 parents sat in a big semicircle, and Pia got up to introduce the demonstration. "I had been introduced to the concept of 'walking music' and taught how to use the auditory motor system in a workshop for therapists in Syracuse, New York," Pia said. "When I came back home, I started using it with Sarah. I put the music on the CD player in the family room and then we went in the hallway. I told her to start walking when she could 'feel' the rhythm in her body. She stood at one end of the hallway and focused for a minute and then took a step forward. Her gait improved immediately: her step length equalized and her limp all but disappeared. I can still see her face lighting up in a smile, as she understood that she could do it."

Then Pia introduced Sarah. She stood up and stepped into the open space, where the group surrounded her, eager to see what would happen next. I asked Sarah to show us what she had learned. Sarah nodded. First she would demonstrate what she called her "sloppy" walk. She walked across the open space, back and forth, with a definite limp.

When she was back beside me, I turned on a recording of the music she had been using with Pia. Sarah paused for a moment, listened intently, and then retraced her steps across the room. But this time, she walked normally.

No limp. No issues with balance. She walked with her arms and legs moving with a reciprocal swinging action. The audience gasped, clapped, and cheered. Sarah's mom burst into tears. It was an amazing moment.

But Sarah wasn't finished. I turned off the CD player and she held up her hand. She said, "Be quiet, please." The room became hushed again. Sarah closed her eyes for a moment and then opened them, and without music, in a silent room in front of a room full of strangers, Sarah repeated her perfect walk, this time without music. When she returned to my side, she looked up at me and then at the roomful of grown-ups. When the applause died down, she explained what had happened.

"I turned the music on in my head."

— • —

I knew that music could improve the walk of a child with cerebral palsy, but Sarah was the first person to show me that *imagined* music could achieve the same result. It was another aha! moment, one that came at the end of a chain of events that began more than a decade earlier with something I saw on TV.

I was flipping through channels one night and stopped when I found a documentary that featured a New Orleans jazz band. The band was playing Dixieland favourites at a seniors' residence. They were in the middle of "When the Saints Go Marching In" when a woman with Alzheimer's disease came into the room. She was dragging a walker along behind her. She was so frail she could barely walk, but she paused in her progress, her attention caught by what she was hearing. Then, she let go of the walker and clapped in time to the beat. And then—and this was the most amazing thing—she danced out of the walker. When the music stopped she stumbled and almost fell to the floor.

Somehow, the familiar tune had triggered something in this woman's brain. An ancient neural map had been reignited, and the dementia and poor motor control that had put her in a walker had briefly disappeared. She danced until the music stopped.

The scene sparked a connection. We all know that we run better and walk with a more consistent pace when listening to music. In fact, it is common knowledge that all kinds of exercise get a boost if performed to music. Think for a moment what would happen if someone turned off the music in the middle of an aerobics class: without the music there would be chaos. A number of research trials have shown that music's effect is backed up by science. One recent study, for example, showed that people recovering from heart surgery who listened to music while they exercised routinely prolonged their workout by as much as 70 percent. "People walking to music with a beat at the speed of their steps have better fitness results than people who do not use music," reported one of the researchers involved in the trial. "And when people listen to music with an amplified beat—sort of like walking to marching music where the walking beat is very strong—these people have even better fitness results than those just walking with regular music."[5] These days, you can order up a personal playlist that matches your choice of music to the tempo of your walk or run, through apps such as RockMyRun and PaceDJ. The International Olympic Committee allows music as a training aid, but bans the use of music from athletic competition: apparently the use of an iPod or MP3 player gives athletes an unfair edge. All this is common knowledge. There's something about music that bypasses other brain circuits.

Would music give a child with a dysfunctional walk a strategy to bypass the habit?

Once the Magee Clinic was up and running, I hired a music therapist, but it didn't help. I hired a dancer to see if we could integrate movement and dance. I had a graduate student working with the Canadian ballet school on another project, and the concept seemed plausible, but somehow nothing we tried quite jelled. Children's songs from *Sesame Street*, for example, were a failure. I thought they would be easy to understand and the beat was catchy. It worked for some and not at all for others. The problem seemed to be that a number of children with early neurologic problems also had auditory-processing issues. For them, the words that went with the songs were confusing. I then tried just a simple beat with a metronome. This was a total failure. Some of the children actually became clumsier. I think that when they tried to match their steps to the fixed beat of the metronome, they found it too rigid and unforgiving, and they were quickly frustrated.

Then I ran into an old friend who was a musician. Greg Adams wrote jingles for advertising campaigns, matching music to the action in the advertisement. I persuaded Greg to help me find a way to use music in treating the children.

Our first attempts had indifferent results as we tried to find the "right" beat to stimulate a better walking pattern. I would walk up and down, mimicking the typical walk of the two main patterns of cerebral palsy, hemiplegia, involving one side of the body, and diplegia, involving both legs. Once Greg had created a walking-music tape, we would try it out at the end of the standardized test of function at each clinic visit. Our experiments did, finally, achieve some success. Greg was one of the first people in Toronto to use a music synthesizer. This new technology allowed him to create complex music with multiple layers of rhythm. We found that the music that worked best had a clearly defined primary beat combined with layered sub-beats. The child would pick out the beat that worked and follow it. It created movement options and had a kind of safety net. The tunes Greg came up with offered 1:4, 1:8, or 1:16 rhythms layered over each other. As long as everything was going along well, the child would continue walking to the chosen beat. However, if he stumbled or lost a step, he could recover by picking up the next available beat.

When I watched a child walk to the music, it was obvious when it was working, when the music was lodged in his brain. It was obvious if he was distracted: he would swerve off course, lose his balance, or become clumsy. Usually, however, he would catch himself, attend to the music again, and walk smoothly.

Once we had developed the right music, we started experimenting with people with other neurologic problems and quickly discovered the positive response could be generalized across other diagnoses. One of our early trials involved a young teenager with an incomplete spinal cord injury. Ashley could walk independently but slowly. By temperament, she was strong-willed, very much her own person, and she had for a long time insisted on walking to and from school by herself. We gave her a CD to listen to while she was walking, and within a week her mother reported that the trek to school, which used to take her daughter twenty-five minutes, now took only eleven. She was faster than she used to be, and more significantly, she now walked with a more balanced and comfortable gait.

— • —

The corticospinal motor system is the primary and most efficient controller of motor movement. When it is damaged, the level and severity of injury determines the resulting neurologic syndrome. Walking or moving in time to music takes advantage of the undamaged parts of the auditory motor system. With practice the individual can learn to access this area for motor processing without requiring the real-time auditory cue. Just remembering the music and its pace can serve as a cue. This approach to rehabilitation is based on the concept of recruiting the undamaged areas of the brain to help accomplish a task, rather than trying only to improve function in the damaged area that normally controls the movement. It is another example of the substitution neuroplasticity described by Paul Bach-y-Rita.

The auditory motor system was the first area where adult brain neurogenesis (the birth of new brain cells) was documented in animals. Fernando Nottebohm, a long-time researcher and professor working at Rockefeller University in New York, came to that conclusion by paying attention to the songs that canaries sing. What he was able to show, in studies dating back to the early 1980s, was that a male canary's brain changes according to the season. In spring, the part of the brain that controls singing actually grows as the male bird makes a maximal effort to attract a mate through song. In summer, when its tunes are no longer needed, that part of the brain shrinks—only to expand again in the fall, when it's time to learn and rehearse something new. The changes to the bird's brain involved the birth and death of thousands of neurons. Nottebohm and his assistants proved that canaries possess adult neuroplasticity.[6]

The auditory motor system is a great example of one of the major limitations of normal science. It is an old adage that scientists only study what they can measure. As a result, the parts of the auditory motor system that are well researched are those parts that control speech production and song. In the study of the human auditory motor system, a quick internet search of academic resources brings up close to a million hits, but they are nearly all related to the perception of sound, the processing of sound, and the production of speech or song, the latter in both animals and man. Yet the association of music with improved motor performance in walking and dance has been known for many years. Oliver Sacks, in his book *Musico-philia*, discusses people with a wide range of disabilities, from Parkinson's disease to Alzheimer's, who have been shown to move better to music.[7] We now know that the response to a rhythmic beat is present early and seems universal to humans. Even babies born prematurely can rapidly entrain the rhythm of their suck to a musical beat with a beneficial effect.[8]

No one knows for sure where the auditory motor system that controls gait resides in the brain, as it is not yet possible to accurately measure what happens in the brain if the subject is moving. Whatever its precise location, the auditory motor system serves as a powerful backup to the primary cortico-spinal system. Just about any activity that has a rhythmic or repetitive component is performed more easily and at a higher level when it is done to music. In the normal individ-ual, walking, running, or dancing to music activates both the corticospinal system and the auditory motor system. The cer-ebellum also contributes to the ability to dance, particularly if the dance routine is rapid or complicated.

The closest investigators have come to studying the motor response to beat has been in experiments conducted by Joyce Chen and her colleagues in Montreal. They found that when subjects tapped their fingers in time to music while undergoing a functional brain scan, their motor cortex, basal ganglia, cerebellum, and interconnections between the auditory and the dorsal premotor cortex all were activated.[9] The important point of this finding is that the auditory areas are rarely damaged in the majority of children with cerebral palsy, and we found a rapid and reliable response to music in most of these children.

Michael Thaut and Gerald McIntosh, founding members of the Neurologic Music Therapy (NMT) group based at Colorado State University, have demonstrated measurable benefit of music to patients with stroke, Parkinson's disease, traumatic brain injury, and cerebral palsy. "Therapists and physicians use music now in rehabilitation in ways that are not only backed up by clinical research findings," they write, "but also supported by an understanding of some of the mechanisms of music and brain function." They also acknowledge, however, that despite the fact the trials to which NMT has been subjected meet the standard demanded by evidence-based science, their findings about its benefits "have not been reflected in public awareness ... or even among some professionals."[10] In both adults and children, the *dancing* brain is able to work with the *walking* brain to change movement patterns.

It's undoubtedly true that there is resistance to accepting music as a form of rehabilitation therapy. For some, it is not enough to know that a particular strategy works if the mechanism that makes it work is not fully understood. For others, the fact that this therapy is not routinely reimbursed by third-party payers may also play a significant role in discouraging use. What we know for certain is that the explanation of the music effect depends on the brain's ability to reorganize and reallocate its resources to maximize function. Bach-y-Rita called it "substitution neuroplasticity," using tactile sensations from the skin of the back and the tongue to compensate for lost balance and sight. The music tapes brought the undamaged auditory motor system into action to improve the damaged motor systems of the child with cerebral palsy.

— • —

I agree with Thaut and McIntosh that auditory motor substitution neuroplasticity is an important mechanism and one that is significantly underused in both adult and pediatric neurorehabilitation. This type of neuroplasticity involves purposefully using a different brain system to restore lost function. There are other well-known examples of substitution neuroplasticity in the rehabilitation of adult stroke or head injury. Aphasia means inability to speak. But many people with aphasia can sing. Speaking and singing are produced by different parts of the brain, and the aphasia in patients with stroke causes damage just in the area responsible for producing speech. If the areas that we use when singing are undamaged, the patient may be able to learn to communicate with words set to music. With lots of practice, the brain can learn to speak without the need to impose a rhythm.

I discovered at a workshop that this technique could also be useful for teenagers who were non-verbal.

The therapists had brought in a thirteen-year-old boy for me to see. He had a severe form of spastic quadriplegia and was essentially non-verbal. He was intelligent and used his communication device well, but his speech was limited to "yes" and "no" and few emotional grunts that his parents and sister could understand. He had moved out of traditional speech therapy years earlier and now only worked with an augmentative communication therapist to improve his speech software. I said it was worth another try, now that he was entering puberty. At this age, the frontal lobes mature. This is important because, thanks to functional brain scanning, scientists had discovered accessory speech centres in the frontal cortex. They had found that there are new areas of the brain that contribute to speech that only become active as the frontal lobes mature during the second peak period of neuroplasticity. This young man was now in puberty and I thought he might also be able to access the newly maturing parts of his brain.

I told him to listen to music—his choice of songs—and to try to first just make noises as he listened. Gradually he might be able to start to sing and from there, the therapists could use the same techniques commonly used with adults after a stroke. Then his sister spoke up: "John can sing." All of us, especially his parents, were shocked. Well, his sister said, "John sang along with everyone else at day camp the previous summer." She had never thought to tell anyone. It turns out that the *singing* brain can also teach the *speaking* brain a new way of working, once all the available brain systems come online during puberty.[11]

— • —

The effect of music and rhythm is amazing, but even therapists who know what music can do often are reluctant to use it. When I first advocated its use, the music player most widely used was the portable CD player, and it was difficult to sync it when you were moving. Another technical issue for many therapists was their work conditions. A typical therapy room is a shared space with up to ten child/parent/therapist interactions going on at once. Clearly, it was hard to introduce music in such a busy, distracting situation. Yet that's not a problem any longer. Now that iPods, MP3 players, cellphones, and comfortable ear buds are widely available, the obstacles to music as a therapeutic device have been mostly eliminated.

It is an inexpensive, effective intervention for most children with cerebral palsy. It may also help children with upper-limb problems perform repetitive tasks with both hands.

Walk with Your Eyes

I stumbled on another way to demonstrate underlying brain strength through luck and desperation at a workshop for therapists. Suzanne Davis Bombria, an experienced neuro-developmental therapist (NDT), hosted the program at her Florida clinic. My first challenge when I find myself in front of a group of therapists is to grab their attention. I want to demonstrate how much positive change is possible and how easily it can be made to happen. I know that they're a little skeptical at first. So my goal, at the outset, is to show them something that will impress them.

The first technique that I demonstrated was with Suzanne's son, Shane, who had cerebral palsy. I asked the therapists to set up tables in two rows. Shane normally walked in a walker but not with good form. A common finding in children who use walkers is that they bear most of their weight on their upper body, leaning forward, taking advantage of the wheels on the walker to move forward. The legs move along, but they aren't taking most of the weight. When Shane walked between the two rows of tables, just putting his hands on the surface for balance, it was a novel, challenging task. It took him out of his habitual way of walking, and suddenly, he straightened up and transferred the work of walking to his legs instead of the arms. It was an impressive change.

Then I tried the same technique with the tables on a different patient. Susan was sixteen or seventeen years old and also walked with a walker. Her diagnosis was moderately severe ataxic quadriplegia, a complex type of cerebral palsy that affects all four limbs. She was weak in all her muscle groups and had major problems with balance. I wanted to see if we could improve her walking by giving her a better balance point. I asked her to walk with her hands just touching the edges of the tables and it worked, sort of. She improved but not much. I was aware that my demonstration was falling flat. There's nothing like a roomful of silent doubters to apply pressure on a speaker who's trying to make an impression. I saw more than one member of the audience glance at her watch. Then I remembered that Susan always looked down watching her feet as she walked, even in the walker. It gave me another idea.

I asked for some masking tape and I had them stick it in a horizontal line at her eye level on the wall at the end of the runway of tables. I told Susan to take her hands off the tables, stare at the tape, and start walking.

She walked perfectly.

When she came to the end of the runway, she turned around and—without the tape to stare at—walked badly again. And then she turned around again and walked perfectly. That tape was magic.

"The change was dramatic," Suzanne, the therapist, said afterwards. "It was effective in getting her taller and more symmetric in her body. It is a strategy that has never left my mind. I have used it many, many times."

— • —

We all know that our fine motor skills and balance improve with visual input. Think of trying to balance on one leg with your eyes shut. Using our eyes improves both balance and ease of movement. When Susan tried to walk, she looked down, watching her feet to try to improve her balance. But this actually made her balance problems worse. For most of us, keeping upright while moving, reaching and grasping an object, or simply maintaining our balance is relatively easy. But these functions all depend on our ability to accurately process different kinds of sensory information. One important input comes from the vestibular system, which consists of three canals located in the inner ear that detect different planes of movement. The vestibular system works best when your head is upright. Susan, by looking at her feet, was making her ataxia worse by knocking out the vestibular system. A visual cue helped keep her oriented in space. With this cue at eye level—the horizontal tape—her head was up and both her vestibular system and her visuomotor system were able to compensate for her cerebellar ataxia. She walked normally. She had better awareness of her surroundings and she could focus more easily on her balance. And because keeping her eye on a visual target was a novel exercise, it took her outside her habit.

While there is little research on the auditory motor system as applied to walking skills, there are many studies on vision. Michael Merzenich and his Posit Science group have produced more than fifty papers showing that training visual awareness, perception, and memory all improve balance and coordination.[12] For older individuals, who may find themselves losing their balance, Posit Science (the online version goes by the name BrainHQ) offers a program of corrective brain-training exercises.[13] The important point, perhaps, is that it's not vision or physical awareness of our position in space or even the intricate workings of the inner ear that keep us balanced—even though all three systems play a role. The crucial element is how the brain functions to integrate the input.

— • —

Numerous brain-training experiments have demonstrated, over and over, that the brain can be encouraged to develop a new habit that replaces a dysfunctional one. These studies also help debunk an old theory—a theory that actually earned its inventors the Nobel Prize for Physiology or Medicine in 1981. David Hubel and Torsten Wiesel were investigating visual function in animals. They found that if a young animal was unable to use its eyes for a period of weeks after birth, its visual system did not develop. From this and other experiments they came up with the hypothesis that there are critical periods in a young animal's life (and by extrapolation, in a child's life too) when the brain develops. When the critical period is over, the game's over. Brain function cannot improve if the animal misses the critical period of development early in life.

For decades, the critical period theory demonstrated in baby animals was applied to baby humans. Amblyopia, commonly known as lazy-eye syndrome, causes a loss of vision in one eye. It occurs in some children with cerebral palsy as well as the able-bodied population. It became accepted dogma that if a child's crossed eye was left untreated over the age of three, the brain learned to shut off the image from the weaker eye and the child became half-blind. A number of studies in the 1980s and 1990s showed that in an older child or adult with amblyopia, sight could be improved with later training, but the improvement was slight and did not have much of a functional effect. Missing the critical period of binocular vision (using both eyes together) in childhood seemed to produce a permanent loss.

Then neuroplasticity came into play. This was a challenge to Torsten Wiesel, a challenge that he handled as a great scientist would. In a commentary in the *Journal of Neurobiology*, he first recapped some of the key studies that led to the

Nobel Prize. "In the early years, David Hubel and I—and perhaps Charles Gilbert as well—had a rather static view of the circuitry of the visual cortex. We firmly believed that once cortical connections were established in their mature form, they stayed in place permanently."[14] Then, when Michael Merzenich and his group published their findings on sensory neuroplasticity, demonstrating that the adult brain could reorganize in response to changed input, Wiesel and Charles Gilbert took a new look at the visual cortex in an adult monkey model. They found that "the adult primary visual cortex is indeed *surprisingly* modifiable in terms of receptive field structure and the unmasking of hitherto hidden connections."[15] In other words, when the critical period ends, the game is not over, as they once thought. In a letter to the editor of *Nature*, Wiesel and Gilbert seemed to reject the original position of Hubel and Wiesel that gave them the Nobel Prize—that the brain is set after the critical period, and embraced the idea that the brain can change, even in adulthood: "The adult brain has a remarkable ability to adjust to changes in sensory input. Removal of afferent input to the somatosensory, auditory, motor or visual cortex results in a marked change of cortical topography."[16] In other words, the adult brain is changeable in response to new inputs. This new information modified the critical period theory that claimed the adult brain was resistant to change.

So, animal brains can change with the right training, but what about older children with amblyopia? These are the children with a crossed or "lazy" eye that either was not treated early or failed to respond to treatment. The crossed eye gives the child double vision. If this situation persists, over the age of approximately three years, the brain turns off the input from the crossed eye and it becomes functionally blind. Early studies had seemed to confirm the critical period theory as later training of the blind eye had little effect.

Researchers at the Research Institute of McGill University Health Centre in Montreal have recently developed a clever, more neuroplastic approach. All the previous attempts to encourage the brain to start using the blind eye had been passive, just temporarily putting a patch over the normal eye. The results of this type of treatment at any age over three years were marginal at best. There was some slight improvement in vision, but depth perception—requiring both eyes to work together—could not be restored. The new McGill neuroplastic technique depended on the assumption that the human visual system also has plasticity and the previous poor results of treatment were more of a *treatment failure* than proof of a visual system critical period. "The key to improving vision for adults, who currently have no other treatment options, was to set up conditions that would enable the two eyes to cooperate for the first time in a given task," Robert Hess, the lead author, told a reporter.[17]

Participants in the study played a version of a video game, Tetris, which requires the player to guide oblong blocks into oblong niches as they fall vertically on the screen. Half of the participants played the game with the weaker eye while the dominant eye was patched. This was one step up from just patching the stronger eye, but it was still a forced-use paradigm. The other half of the subjects played dichoptically, meaning that each eye was able to view only one part of the game. Both eyes *had* to work together in order to position the blocks. The dichoptic group showed dramatically improved vision in the weaker eye as well as better 3-D depth perception. The participants who played with the strong eye covered, meanwhile, had only modest improvement—until they, too, had undergone the dichoptic drill.[18] Just working with the weak eye, like working with the abnormal walk, had limited success. The brain loves a novel challenge. When the subjects had to use both eyes to play the game, the brain took up the challenge and figured out a way to make it work.

These results went completely against the critical period concept. The subjects were able to both strengthen the weak side and improve their depth perception, which requires both eyes to work together. This is just one more example of an established idea that needs to be updated as a result of new observations and research studies. The concept of critical periods in development is also a classic example of the dangers inherent in extrapolating the results of an animal experiment to a human child. Clearly there are *sensitive periods* in development, when it is easier to forge the correct connections, but our complex brains are not rigid. They are adaptable and respond best to novelty, challenge, and consequences.

The challenge of learning a second language is a good example of the importance of sensitive periods. Early exposure makes all the difference. In certain areas of Switzerland, where children routinely hear several languages throughout their childhood, it is not unusual for a child to develop fluency in two, three, or even four languages. And yet, those of us who have attempted to master another language later in life know how difficult it can be. Difficult, but using modern brain-training software, many more adults are able to become reasonably fluent in a new language. The point is that our brains are learning machines. If we can figure out how to present the material in the right way, and at the right time, change happens. This offers real hope for children with early brain or nerve injury to literally rewire their brains.

— • —

Substitution neuroplasticity involves using an intact brain centre to stand in for another area that is damaged. Both the auditory and the visual motor circuits offer an opportunity for a therapist to develop a new habit that replaces one that is dysfunctional. It would be wonderful if substitution neuroplasticity worked all the time, but that's not what happens. Sometimes you have to experiment, reach deep into the toolbox of techniques and technologies to come up with something new. Sometimes nothing works.

Non-responders may not yet have enough recovered brain to perform the action. They may need to mature a bit more before they can learn how to bring in help from the rest of their brain. Creating awareness of possibility can be the first step, teaching the brain that more is possible. Different paths may lead to unexpectedly positive results.

nine

The Girl Who Forgot Her Hand

We now know that some children can recover from a brain injury. The problem is that while their brains are still in the process of healing and maturing, they develop maladaptive movement patterns. These movement patterns become comfortable for the child, and remain in place even after the brain has recovered to the point where more efficient movements are possible. A habit has been established, and it can hide evidence of brain recovery.

The question, then, is this: How can these habits be replaced with new ones? As I searched for the answer to this question, some important clues came from outside my professional silo, from the world of nerve damage. It turned out that the treatment of an early brain injury that produces cerebral palsy had a few things in common with the treatment of peripheral nerve injury. In both cases, the question we faced was, Can you develop normal function after the brain (or the nerve) has healed? If so, how?

——— • ———

In the Neonatal ICU, infants are closely monitored in the early days of life, and in mid-1970s when I was a neonatal fellow, we had to take arterial blood samples—a lot of them, sometimes for a period of weeks. The blood samples were very small, but even so, taking blood from a preterm, low birthweight baby was challenging. We took some of the samples from the brachial artery, a major artery in the upper arm, but if the needle hit the median nerve right beside the artery, the child's ability to manipulate objects with the affected hand could be impaired.

In babies treated in 1974, we found a variable degree of peripheral median nerve damage in eighteen children seen in the Follow-Up Clinic. They could not grasp a small object as most of us do, by bringing thumb and index finger together. The thumb tended to stay unmoving, in a neutral position, and the index finger was held straight out. This was the classic "pointing index finger" of median nerve damage.

We wrote an article to alert doctors and nurses to the danger of damaging the nerve.[1] When the children were between eighteen months and two years old, I tested them with the clinic occupational therapist, Sarah Forsythe. I picked this age to test their function as by then we expected that any nerve recovery that was possible would be completed. So, we got down on a mat with the children to see if we could get them to use their thumb and index finger in play. They had all learned to use their third, fourth, and little fingers to manipulate objects and pick up small items. They got to be pretty good at it, but it clearly wasn't ideal.

In retrospect, what we did was obvious. We pinned the sleeve of the children's good hand to their top, so they couldn't move that hand, and we taped together the three fingers of the impaired hand, which the children had been using to pick things up. We scattered treats, like M&Ms and raisins, on the mat in front of them. If they wanted to get the treats from mat to mouth, they had to figure out how to grasp them in a way that was new to them. Clumsily at first, but with increasing dexterity, they managed to bring the index finger and thumb together with enough pressure to grasp and hang on to the treats.

Our strategy worked. We made them use their non-functional fingers. If they could make just one pincer grasp, then we knew that their median nerve had regenerated. The reality that they preferred to use the outer three fingers to pick up objects was an early-learned habit acquired before the median nerve had recovered. Habit hides recovery, just as it did in the boy who could run but not walk.

We had proved that the nerve had recovered, but how could we get them to use the normal pincer grasp on a regular basis instead of their work-around method, using the outer three fingers?

The answer came later from Edward Taub, a behavioural neuroscientist from Atlanta. His solution would open the door to a new way of treating not only patients with peripheral nerve damage, but also patients with cerebral palsy.

In the 1980s, Taub and his associates designed a series of experiments with monkeys to study what happens when the link between the brain and the limb is altered for a period of time. First they cut the sensory nerves so that the monkey couldn't feel anything from that limb. Initially the monkeys tried to keep using it, but they lost their balance and fell, or they dropped food items and went hungry. After a while, they used the other limb to do the job. It didn't take long before the monkeys were exclusively using the better limb while the other one was left hanging. Taub called it "learned non-use."[2]

Then Taub set out to see if he could reverse the effects. Once the sensory nerve injury had recovered, he bound up the good limb to immobilize it. Now the monkeys either had to use the neglected limb or they would be unable to feed themselves, move about, or carry out a large part of their normal daily activities. Sure enough, with this challenge, he found that the monkeys were able to recover the use of the neglected limb. He called this "forced-use," but soon revised the term to the less threatening "Constraint-Induced Movement Therapy," or CIMT.[3]

It took a considerable amount of time and practice for the animal to overcome the learned non-use, though.[4] If he took the constraint off too soon, the animal just went back to using the stronger side. Why? During the time of nerve injury, the brain had developed powerful circuits to control the limb that was taking over. Those circuits were so strong that they kept working, even when the constraints came off the limb. It shows why it's so hard to drop a bad habit: the brain's circuit that's running the old habit still wants to do its job, even when you learn something new. The same thing happens when a child with cerebral palsy learns a more functional walk in a therapy session. Obviously the new pattern can be learned, but it is not yet strong enough to persist, so the child falls back into his well-established habit on the way home after a therapy session.

Taub and his colleague Steven Wolf went on to refine protocols for CIMT in a clinical setting, working first with adults who'd had a stroke. He put a mitt on the hand or a sling on the arm of individuals who had lost the use of their arm and hand on one side. Then he gave them purposeful tasks to practise intensively for extended periods. Here he was combining his concept of restraint with the idea of purposeful training.[5] With a mitt on their unaffected hand, the test subjects might be required to pick up pennies and put them in a piggy bank, or shift canned goods and dishes from one shelf to another. Whereas standard rehabilitation requires the patient to attend a clinic two or three times a week for an hour at a time, Taub and Wolf's regime required continuous training for six or more or hours a day, over a period of ten days or two weeks or longer. From the start the experiments yielded positive results and CIMT is now used widely in adult stroke rehabilitation.

Taub's clinic at the University of Alabama has since developed extensive training protocols based on this idea to treat a number of conditions, including traumatic brain injury, brain tumours, and multiple sclerosis.[6] But here was the part that I found really exciting: Taub found that CIMT worked for another condition—cerebral palsy.[7]

— • —

Fortunately, few, if any, children now experience a median nerve injury. Oxygen levels are now routinely measured non-invasively through the skin. However, another peripheral nerve injury, brachial plexus injury, is as frequent as cerebral palsy, affecting two to four per thousand live births, with wide regional variations. The brachial plexus is a network of nerves that transmits signals from the spine to the shoulder, arm, and hand.[8] It can be damaged by trauma at birth, most commonly with a difficult breech delivery or an arrest of delivery with the shoulder of the baby becoming stuck in the birth canal. The injury is diagnosed shortly after birth when the child's arm is noticed to be hanging loosely, with little, if any, movement. Luckily, in a high proportion of cases, the injury is only a stretch (like a bruise) of the nerve and the arm starts moving within a few weeks. The others, roughly 25 percent of infants with this injury, have a continuing problem.

The children with persisting weakness, even those with a very mild injury, often have problems with the growth of the arm and hand, bone and joint distortions, and decreased function.[9] It is commonly accepted that peripheral nerve injuries have a generally good potential for recovery, but in many children, even though the nerves had recovered, their functional abilities using the arm had not.

Why?

After seeing a great many of these cases at the Magee Clinic, I asked Alan McComas at McMaster University to help sort out this puzzle. Alan and his associates studied sixteen children age four to fourteen with BPI. Their nerves connecting their spinal cord to their hands were fine. Yet none of them were able to lift their arm above the shoulder, and most had significant weakness extending from their shoulder and forearm all the way down to the hand.

So what was happening? This was in the late 1990s, and the Nobel Prize–winning common wisdom from Hubel and Wiesel was that there was a critical period for learning in early childhood. The problem, McComas decided, was that by the time their BPI network of nerves had recovered, it was too late for the children to learn how to use their hand and fingers. The children had missed the window of opportunity. McComas put it in scientific language: "The impairment is a form of developmental apraxia [or non-use] caused by defective motor programming in early infancy."[10] At this time, missing a critical period of development was thought to produce a permanent loss.

Our article—my name was on it too—was published as the lead article in *Neurology*, which is the main scholarly journal for neurologists. In the same issue, though, was another study by a French group of investigators who had come to a different conclusion.

The French surgeons had repaired the injured nerves of the brachial plexus in little children age two to four, but it didn't turn out the way they expected. The surgery was supposed to help the children bring their hands to their mouths, but instead it did the opposite—the children developed elbow extension. When the children tried to use the arm, it was held out straight instead of bending. They had a stiff arm.

It was an odd situation. The investigators knew the biceps nerve had recovered—the connection was there on

EMG testing—but the children had no notion how to access it. They had never learned how to flex the elbow. They had what we called a developmental apraxia, or non-use.

The French doctors came up with an innovative solution. They put botulinum toxin (in this case it was Botox) into the over-firing triceps muscle on the back of the arm, two or three times over a period of eight to twelve months. This weakened the triceps muscle for a prolonged period of time. At the same time, they actively exercised the biceps muscle to create elbow flexion, hoping that the children would learn how to do elbow flexion while the triceps was temporarily weakened.

Before the injection of botulinum, when the children tried to move their arm, the strong triceps muscle would respond first and quickly overpower the weaker biceps muscle. However, the combination of weakening the strong triceps and exercising the weak biceps muscle changed all that. The children gradually developed normal reciprocal movement at the elbow, wiring a new pattern of movement into their brains and overcoming their developmental non-use. By the end of a year of Botox treatment, they had a normally functioning elbow with flexion and extension and required no further injections.[11]

The contrast between the Canadian and the French studies was striking. Both the Canadian and the French teams were dealing with the same problem—children whose injured nerves had healed, one spontaneously and one with the help of surgery. In both cases, the children had never learned how to use the recovered nerve function. There the similarities ended. The Canadian team did not think there was a viable treatment option because the children had not learned to use their fingers properly during the all-important critical period of development. The French surgeons, on the other hand, had found a way to fix it.

The editors of *Neurology* understood this. In a short editorial, they noted that the French surgeons had demonstrated convincingly not only that the nerves were intact, but also that the maladaptive movement could be fixed. How? The problem was not in the nerves—in an "aberrant peripheral regeneration," they noted. Instead, the problem was a "central abnormality." It was, in other words, in the brain. The Botox injections worked by allowing the children to flex their elbows, which in turn rewired their brains. Or, as the *Neurology* editors put it, "The more normal movement allowed by the injections produced activity dependent plasticity that eliminated the central abnormality or cancelled its functional effect."[12]

This was Michael Merzenich's activity-dependent neuroplasticity in action, and the same mechanism can be used to help children with early brain and nerve damage.

— • —

Sometimes you don't need a shot of Botox or a restraint to uncover the recovery of the nerve that has been hidden under layers of bad habits. Jenna is a bright little girl who had a brachial plexus injury at birth. Immediately after the injury, Jenna's arm was paralyzed and this lasted for months. As the nerve gradually recovered, she used only those muscle groups that recovered first and ignored the ones that were not working. Her brain wired in the pattern of using only some of her muscles. As the abnormal movement pattern was repeated, thousands of times, it became her habitual movement. Jenna's abnormal arm lift halfway up was an early-learned habit that was automatic to her.

She started in therapy with Pia Stampe when she was three years old. Early treatment for brachial plexus injury is highly variable, and many children do not qualify for early intervention programs. "At the start," Pia said, "she could not lift her arm up at all. She was not activating the muscles around her wrist or elbow very well. There was a lot of weakness." Pia put Jenna on TES for a couple of months to get some muscle growth, and then used EMG-triggered stimulation to activate the muscles to the point where she could also do resistance and functional training.

By age six, Jenna could lift her arm to about eighty degrees, just about shoulder height, but no higher. Then, on the spur of the moment, Pia asked her to do something new—jumping jacks. All of a sudden, Jenna's arm came way up over her head. Here was a girl who couldn't lift her arm above her shoulder, but when she did jumping jacks, she had a full range of movement. It was an incredible sight. Her nerves had obviously healed, but we didn't see it because her early habit of lifting her arm up only halfway was hiding the actual extent of her recovery.

The explanation was simple: an early-learned habit hid her recovered nerve function. But doing jumping jacks was new, and because it was new, it didn't activate the habit. She was helped by momentum—jumping and flinging her arms in the air—but even so, she was actively elevating her arm higher above her shoulder, a skill that seemed to be impossible when she was asked to lift her arm. It was a huge moment for Jenna, and a big opportunity for Pia to help her regain the everyday use of her arm. As a child recovering from a brachial plexus injury, she had already passed the first stage—her nerve had recovered. Now she had to overcome the challenge of developmental non-use and learn to voluntarily lift her arm above her shoulder. We now knew she could; she did the jumping jacks. But she had to learn how to do it every day. It takes time and practice and often we have to wait for brain maturity to assess the full extent of recovery from an injury. Fortunately, the child's brain continues to grow and mature, allowing new functions. All our brains can reorganize and learn new skills into middle age and even later. The challenge in the child with BPI is to recognize the role of both developmental non-use and habit by carefully watching for occasional use of the weaker muscle groups. Once you catch them doing it right, as we did when we saw Jenna do her jumping jacks, you know that the more normal movement patterns can be trained and the muscles strengthened.

———— ◆ ————

Some children do not respond as well as others to an intervention. In some, the problem may be in the brain or due to incomplete nerve recovery, but in many cases the problem relates to body alignment. Body distortion often contributes to the difficulties of children with an early-acquired brain, nerve, or spinal cord injury. It's a significant problem. If the body is distorted or the joints are out of position, improved function is not possible. This is as true for the child with cerebral palsy or BPI as it is for a peak-performance athlete. In human bodies, good function follows good form. The major culprit in children with cerebral palsy is unbalanced muscle pull. In cerebral palsy, the unbalanced pull is caused by progressive spasticity. Over the years, I've come to the conclusion that a significant part of this progressive spasticity is a habit. And, as a habit, much of it can be prevented, and still more can be effectively treated, as we will see in the next chapter.

ten

A New Theory of Spasticity in Children

The most common outward sign of cerebral palsy is spasticity, the exaggerated reflexes and tight muscles that can cause the hand of child with cerebral palsy to clench into a fist and his knees to knock together as he walks on the balls of his feet. Roughly 80 percent of children with CP develop progressive spasticity over the first two to four years of life. Where in the body they encounter the problem can vary. Thirty-nine percent of children have muscle tightness on one side of their bodies. Thirty-eight percent are affected in both legs. The last 23 percent of children have difficulties with both arms and legs.[1]

The outcome for children with spasticity has improved significantly since I was a resident in pediatrics, when most of the children with CP had the most serious form of it. Now,

80 percent of them can walk independently or with a walking aid and have mild to moderate CP.

But can their lives be even better? Now that we know the baby brain can change and heal, can spasticity be fixed?

The traditionalists say no. They contend that CP is caused by brain damage before the age of two to three years, and that irreversible brain damage causes physical problems like spasticity that are irreversible too. Yet for me, the traditional explanation doesn't make sense. We now know that the initial brain injury in babies is reversible. Why should we not assume that the common problem of spasticity is reversible too? I have spent a lot of my professional life as a neonatologist and clinical neuroscientist trying to answer this question, and that inquiry has led me to a new theory of spasticity that offers real hope to children and even adults with cerebral palsy.

Unlike the traditionalists, I think that much of the spasticity in cerebral palsy is a habit, a brain and body habit. As a habit, it can be replaced, just as a wonky tennis serve or an errant golf swing can be changed. It takes time. It takes persistent work. It may require medications and surgery, but it can be done. I have found that much of spasticity is not the inevitable and irreversible effect of irreversible brain damage. It can be improved in most children and adults and even prevented in some at-risk babies, but first you need to understand a bit more about the types of brain damage that now result in the signs and symptoms of spastic cerebral palsy and the natural history of this spasticity as it develops in the infant and toddler.

What Type of Brain Damage
Causes Cerebral Palsy?

The characteristic impairment of movement and posture that we call cerebral palsy begins with a wide variety of underlying brain injuries or problems that interfere with normal brain development. Cerebral palsy can be caused by a brain infection, while the baby is still in the uterus or after birth, in the perinatal period or in the first few years of life. It can be caused by a traumatic birth, causing a bleed in the brain, or by shaken baby syndrome later in life. A significant number of children with cerebral palsy have abnormal brain development early in gestation that affects a variable amount of the brain. Whatever the cause, the timing of the injury to the brain makes a big difference in the physical problems that result.

When a baby has brain damage just before, during, or shortly after birth, we can see, with advanced brain scans, the location and the extent of the damage. This allows us to make predictions about the type of movement problems that a child with an otherwise normal brain may develop. A brain lesion on one side may develop into hemiplegia, a type of cerebral palsy that affects motor control on one side of the body. Brain lesions in both sides of the deep white matter of the brain in premature babies affect the motor control of both legs, which we call diplegia. Damage to both sides of the brain that affects all four limbs is called quadriplegia.

These are the three typical patterns of CP. The severity of impairment in cerebral palsy may range from mild to extremely severe. Some have only the slightest of motor disturbances; others have co-existing problems of cognition, seizures, vision, and hearing as well.

When Can CP Be Diagnosed?

As we have seen, some children with brain damage at birth recover completely. Others do not, but it takes time for one of the three typical patterns of CP to develop. The cerebral palsy traditionalists say they can't make a *confident* diagnosis of cerebral palsy until the child is age three or four, when the characteristic symptoms of CP have developed.[2]

I think their views are shaped by the fact that many of the specialists do not see children with CP until they are referred to a clinic at three to six years old. By this age, the children have clearly established patterns of spasticity. In some children with the more severe forms of cerebral palsy, the early signs of secondary body distortion are already present. The traditionalists, then, only see the children relatively late in the progression of spastic cerebral palsy. As a result, many of them still cling to concept of a permanent disturbance of movement and posture, so they lower their goal to maintaining the level of disability and preventing further deterioration.

Neonatologists like me, on the other hand, see babies with brain damage at birth. We are trained to see the site and severity of damage in the baby brain on brain scans. This early view gives us a different perspective. First, as neonatologists we know that some of the children with early brain damage will show no motor or cognitive problems later on. Their brains will recover completely.[3] We don't know, at this early stage, whether a child will develop CP, but we can identify most of those at risk of developing CP. We can also recognize the very early signs of CP. This is tremendously important: if you can see the early signs, you can move more quickly to prevent problems later in life.

What Are the Early Signs of CP?

In the Neonatal ICU, most survivors of early brain injury initially have muscle weakness and are floppy after discharge. They have been seriously ill and they need time to recover. You can start to first see the telltale signs of CP in the most severely injured babies by three to six months. For the most part, these are babies born at or near full term who had severe asphyxia causing diffuse brain damage. They may also be very complicated preterm infants who suffered repeated brain insults over a period of months. These infants can look surprising normal on the first examination, but the signs of spasticity develop rapidly over the first year of life. I remember seeing a baby in hospital who was born at twenty-six weeks with a brain injury. Mike was weak and floppy at the time of his discharge home, but otherwise looked okay, surprisingly good in fact. Twelve months later, he had severe quadriplegic cerebral palsy affecting all four limbs. He was small but proportional at the time of his discharge, but in the following year his brain and skull had hardly grown at all. He now had obvious microcephaly. His movements were spastic and seemed painful. The signs and symptoms of CP had set in with a vengeance.

For infants with less-serious damage, their floppy low tone persists for a variable period of time. The infants with damage on only one side of the brain can often be detected earliest as they use the unaffected arm normally, bringing the hand to mouth and starting to explore the world with the one hand, while the affected arm just lies on the bed. In infants born prematurely with bilateral brain injury deep in the periventricular white matter (PVL), the first sign of problems is often stiffening of the legs, usually about the age of six months. Sometimes, these early problems resolve completely and there is no movement impairment on later examinations. In others, who ultimately are diagnosed with mild to moderate levels of CP, the stiffness and exaggerated reflexes so characteristic of cerebral palsy gradually worsen over the first two to three years of life.

Why Does the Body Deteriorate When the Brain Is Recovering and Growing?

The development of spasticity in the first years of life is, when you think about it, a first-class anomaly. The brains of babies who have suffered brain injury are not only growing rapidly, they are in the process of recovery from the injury. There is no way to tell at present how much they are going to recover, and we do not know how long it takes, but from what we know about how adults recover from strokes, we can assume the recovery takes three to four years. So why do babies and young children begin to experience movement problems in these years, just when their brains are recovering? By definition, the brain injuries and problems that precede cerebral palsy are one-time events. So, despite the fact that the injured brain is in the process of recovery and is growing rapidly, the body is starting on the road of progressive impairment of movement and spasticity.

It's a mystery that urgently needs to be solved. To begin with, let's look at the basic facts:

First, everyone agrees that cerebral palsy is caused by a one-time brain problem and the brain injury does not get worse. It is, by definition, a non-progressive brain disorder. The brain either stays the same or has some degree of recovery.

Second, baby brains develop over a prolonged time period with ballistic brain growth and maturation in two periods, from birth to four to six years and again during puberty. During these periods of explosive growth, the brain matures and new capabilities come online.

Third, spasticity is the most common outward sign of cerebral palsy, occurring in up to 80 percent of children with CP. The brain injury and spasticity are causally linked, but as the child's brain matures and recovers, the spasticity becomes worse, not better. The linked signs of brain damage and spasticity go in different directions. The brain is either staying the same or getting better, but the spasticity and body distortion get worse as the child grows.

What's going on? Let's take a closer look at what happens when a baby with brain damage tries to move, and how that differs from a child without brain injury.

How Babies Learn to Move

The way the brain controls the muscles in the body is the result of a complicated but beautiful design. When it's working, it's invisible, as is all great design. The child learns to walk fluidly and doesn't have to think about it.

Consider the way a baby learns to move. When the baby wants to bring his fingers to his mouth, the brain tells the muscles to move, and the muscles respond in a balanced reciprocal manner. To raise the hand to mouth, the arm flexors on the inside of the arm contract while the arm extensor muscles on the outside relax. If both sets of muscles work at the same time, the arm gets stuck in mid position. After a while, the baby's hand and fingers make it to his mouth smoothly. You can see how it works for yourself if you bring your hand to your mouth. Feel your biceps (on the front of your arm) as you do. You'll feel the muscle tighten. Now, as you do the same hand-to-mouth movement, feel the back of your arm. The muscle should feel loose. That's how muscles about a joint work. As one muscle activates, the other muscle relaxes. It's a beautifully coordinated, reciprocal dance of the muscles.

What Happens When a Child with CP Learns to Move

In the child with brain damage, the signal from the brain to activate the muscle is a lot weaker and not normally coordinated. The muscles that respond most easily to the first weak signals from the injured baby brain are the muscles that are inherently stronger. When a baby tries to move his hand to his mouth, the first muscles to respond are the flexor muscles in the upper limbs. These are the muscles that grasp and pull the arms into the chest. With each signal from the brain, these stronger muscles contract and pull the wrist into a flexed position with a fisted hand. After a while, these flexor muscles turn into real bullies. They get tighter while their partners, the muscles that are supposed to relax, do nothing. The muscles that normally extend the wrist and fingers to open and lift the hand up become longer and weaker.

It's not a reciprocal, balanced dance conducted by the brain. The bullies are stomping on the dance floor; their partner muscles are like jilted wallflowers at a high school prom.

Then the child tries to get up. As the child grows and starts to activate the legs purposefully at five to six months of age, the first muscles to fire are the extensor muscles in the lower limbs that hold the body in an upright position. When the toddler tries to stand, the muscles on the back of his leg will tighten, pulling the foot up onto the toes. As this is repeated over and over, the muscles on the front of the leg become will become longer and weaker. The muscles in the front of the leg eventually get so weak that the child will lose the ability to pull the toes up.

In both the upper and lower muscle groups, the abnormal non-reciprocal muscle movements become the *normal* way that body works. The children develop abnormal body habits that we call the characteristic patterns of cerebral palsy.

The Negative Feedback Loop

Once the bully muscles are in command, they set up networks in the brain to consolidate their dominant position and make sure the weaker partner muscles, the ones that are supposed to relax every time the extensor or flexor muscles tighten, are immobilized. It's a negative feedback loop that makes it easy for the brain to fire up the spastic bully muscles and inhibit their opposite partners, which just get weaker. The bullies have not only taken command of the dance floor, but they've also told the band what music to play.

Our brains use a very high proportion of all the energy produced by our bodies. In order to deal with this energy drain, our brains have evolved into efficiency machines. Whatever we repeatedly do, our brain will learn to do better.

Hebb's concept of "neurons that fire together wire together" describes this change. As a nerve network or circuit is fired, over and over, we now know that there are multiple changes that act together to make the process more efficient.

New connections (synapses) between nerve cells are made and strengthened. The neurons learn to fire with less and less input. The neuroscience term for this is that they become *facilitated* circuits. But this is not the only change. Once a facilitated network or circuit fires off, the impulse is carried from the brain all the way down to the muscle on axons. These crucial parts of the system are covered in myelin, which acts like insulation around an electrical wire. As a brain network becomes facilitated, the myelin builds up around the axons arising from it, allowing faster and faster transmission of the brain messages.

So, in the normal situation, there is balanced reciprocal activation and relaxation of our muscles that allows smooth execution of movement. In children with spastic cerebral palsy, there is unbalanced firing of muscle pairs that favours the flexor muscles in the upper limbs and extensor muscles in the lower limbs. Each time a spastic muscle fires, it becomes easier to fire the next time. In addition, each time it fires, it actively inhibits its antagonist non-spastic muscle. A negative feedback loop has been set up and it has become an abnormal brain and body habit.

Growth Makes It Worse

I assume that brain recovery, to whatever extent is possible, is completed by age three to four years. The child has learned to move in whatever way he can, and this abnormal walking pattern has become his *normal* walking pattern. The primary brain injury does not recur, but a negative feedback loop has been set up between the facilitated circuit in the brain and the unbalanced muscles it controls. This negative feedback loop is activated and becomes stronger each time the child moves. Spasticity, in other words, is triggered by brain injury. But it's perpetuated by the negative feedback loop between the muscles and the brain. It's a bad habit, not a sign of ongoing brain damage.

Just to complicate things, the spasticity gets worse every time the child has a growth spurt. The first major growth period is in the first two to four years of life. Children grow to half their adult height by age two to four years. After this ballistic growth period, the child keeps growing but at a less headlong pace. Intermittent growth spurts happen during this time, and parents of children with cerebral palsy soon learn that their child's muscles tighten up during each of these mini-growth spurts. The second period of ballistic growth comes with puberty. By this point, the spastic muscles are firmly in charge, and there is a clear imbalance in the muscles when they move against gravity. During each of the key growth spurts, the rapid progression of muscle imbalance can distort the growth of bone and joints.

Teenagers go through some of the same problems of brain growth and maturation and complicating body growth as found in the very young child. Teenage brains are not growing much in size, but their brains are developing fast. It has been estimated that the teenage brain develops an additional 40 percent of brainpower during puberty. Yet this is the very time that the teenager with cerebral palsy may have a further deterioration in his body's functional abilities. A teenage boy who is able to walk well in the community with forearm crutches as he enters puberty is often only able to do short-term walking in the house by the time he stops growing. In Chapter 13, I will discuss why this occurs so frequently and how to prevent it.

This deterioration in body function is another first-class anomaly: the children's brains are maturing and developing new functional abilities and yet their bodies are getting worse. It doesn't add up if you believe the traditional story that CP is caused by brain damage. If you buy into this line of thinking, you'd expect a better brain to create a better body, or if the body were declining, you would assume it's because the brain is declining. But that's not the case. Body and brain seem to be going in opposite directions yet again. Why?

At the Magee Clinic I had the opportunity to re-examine a large number of children whom I had originally followed for the first three to four years of their life in the Neonatal

Follow-up Program at HSC. This was an incredible experience. I knew what their abnormal tone felt like and how
they moved early in life. It was a real surprise to see them as
teenagers, and what I found then led me to another important
insight. As the children grew through puberty, their spastic
tone increased, yet the extent of the change varied not only
with the severity of their initial brain injury but also directly
with their body type and velocity of growth.

I saw one set of fraternal twins, born prematurely, who
had very a similar degree of brain injury in the neonatal
period. Their brain scans were nearly interchangeable: both
had bilateral periventricular leukomalacia (PVL), which is
damage to the white matter of the brain in the area just next
to the central ventricles of the brain. This is one of the most
common types of damage seen in babies born early, and
I expected the twins to develop spastic diplegia. When I had
last seen them, about three years of age, they both had a mild
degree of spastic diplegia, affecting both legs. Their degree
of impairment was similar when I discharged them from the
Follow-Up Clinic, but by mid puberty when I saw them again,
they were very different.

The boy was tall, muscular, and big boned and it was
clear that he would need orthopedic surgery to correct a progressive crouch gait. He walked independently but with an
unsteady gait and bent knees. His sister was shorter, light
boned, and definitely not as well muscled, and she was basically unchanged in terms of tone and body alignment. She
walked well with a bit of an in-toeing gait, but she was reasonably independent. The difference between the twins was

striking. I started to look more closely at the body type and the expected growth rate of preteens, and over a few years I discovered that the progress of spasticity in puberty was invariably worse in heavily muscled, fast-growing boys than it was in lightly muscled, slower-growing girls.

This insight is extremely important and generally overlooked in the design of most pediatric rehabilitation research trials. Body type, gender, and growth rate are important variables, yet I have never found a study that adequately controls the effect of these variables in the growing teenager with cerebral palsy.

It now seems obvious that the same mechanism—the negative feedback loop—that explains the onset of spasticity as the child begins to grow in the first years of life also explains why spasticity worsens again when a child enters the awkward teenage years. Exactly the same forces are at work.

Spasticity in a child is in many ways harder to deal with than in an adult after a stroke or another form of brain injury. In an infant, uncontrolled spasticity can distort the body as the child grows. In the presence of unequal muscle pull, both muscles and tendons grow differently. The rapid growth rate in the presence of unequal muscle pull also causes bony distortions and, in some, dislocation of major joints, most commonly the hip. Second, because the toddler lacks any memory or awareness of normal movement, he's faced with the challenge of learning something he has never done. All movement is a new skill to be learned and practised, and unfortunately, the maladaptive strategy comes most easily.

An adult who has had a stroke, on the other hand, has a normally grown body, so the spasticity will not distort her body as much. For the adult, who has a memory of what is lost, it is a matter of recovering function. The result is that spasticity looks very different in a child than it does in an adult, even if it's caused by a similar kind of brain injury. Yet either way, it can be treated.

— • —

Treating Spasticity

There are many effective treatments that work at different ages and stages, from the first few months of life to adulthood. I now understand that real improvement in spasticity management depends on doing the right thing, at the right time, and in the right order. In the young toddler, the primary goal is to minimize or even prevent the creation of the negative feedback loop. In the next chapter I will discuss just how easy this is to accomplish, if you actually work with the baby early on. If the negative feedback loop has established itself, a variety of interventions can minimize its effects.

Novel Tasks

The quickest way to take the child out of habit and out of the negative feedback loop that we call spasticity is to get him to do a novel task.

Ask the boy who can't walk properly to run. Ask the girl who can't lift her arms above her shoulders to do jumping jacks. Turn the music on and get the teen dancing. It can produce amazing results because the new task forces the brain to do something new and in the process starts to create a new neural network that instructs the brain to dance, or do jumping jacks, or play soccer. With practice and repetition, the brain will ignore the negative feedback loop that has enabled the bully muscles to impair the body's movement. In time, the negative feedback loop, unused, will fade away.

Water Exercise

Water exercise can produce amazing results, as any elite athlete recovering from injury will tell you. For the child or adult with cerebral palsy, the water removes the negative effect of gravity. When they are free to move without gravity, the bully muscles of a child with CP lose the power they exert on land. With a neutral buoyancy device like the Wet Vest, we can both support the core muscles and keep the child or adult upright in the water. It doesn't take long, only a few minutes, to see the result. A child with diplegia who walks on his toes with knees together on the ground gets into the water, vest on, and after an awkward start, he'll start to move fluidly in the water, in just a few minutes. A teen with hemiplegia will quickly discover that he has to use both arms and legs reciprocally to move forward in the water. If he relies on the old spastic pattern of depending upon the better-functioning side, he will just be able to go around in circles. Our brains love a challenge, and it always surprises me to see just how quickly the old negative feedback loop can be bypassed in the out-of-gravity environment.

This same out-of-gravity principle is also used in many available robotic treadmill gait-training devices. The robotic

shell and/or a gravity-reducing harness force the brain to
figure out a new way of moving, revealing brain recovery
and allowing the repetitive practice that creates a new brain–
body habit.

Botulinum Toxin for Spasticity

Botox is one commonly used medication to treat established,
progressive spasticity. The scientific name is botulinum toxin,
best known as both a deadly food-borne bacteria and a cosmetic treatment for wrinkles. Initially resisted and feared by
physicians, therapists, and parents, it has now been used to
treat progressive spasticity for roughly twenty years. Unfortunately, it is approved for use only in children over the age
of two years.

Physicians inject the medication into the spastic muscle,
where it blocks the muscle from responding to the overactive facilitated circuits firing from the brain. This is the bully
muscle in the negative feedback loop. The high-tone spastic
muscle is temporarily weakened, allowing a time window
to teach the child how to move in a more functional pattern.
Ideally, the tight spastic muscle can now be more effectively
stretched while the inhibitory nerve signals to the opposite
muscle are lessened. In a systematic review of research trials
in cerebral palsy, Botox was awarded the highest approval
rating. Numerous randomized controlled trials have proven
that interrupting the negative feedback loop at the level of
the spastic muscle is effective in CP.[4] Most randomized controlled trials test just one intervention against routine therapy.
In this experimental design, Botox has been clearly shown

to work. However, Botox is addressing just one part of the spastic feedback loop and the effect is relatively short-lived. As soon as the Botox effect wears off, the bully muscles spring back into action and re-establish the negative feedback loop.

Good therapists have learned that a Botox injection lasts longer and produces a better result if the joints are mobilized and the non-spastic antagonist muscles are both activated and strengthened during the time period that the spastic muscles are quieted down. This is the same protocol used by the French therapists to correct the pseudo-spasticity that developed in children with brachial plexus injury post-surgery.[5] The problem in clinical practice is that far too often a physician injects the drug and the child's therapy team is not given notice in time to plan an intensive retaining and strengthening program. The regular frequency of once- or twice-a-week therapy will fail to establish a new habit. Every athlete understands that focused, intensive practice is what builds new habits. They understand that it takes weeks to make a new habit.

Baclofen Pumps

Baclofen pumps were first used for the treatment of spasticity in adult patients with spinal cord injury. They worked very well. More recently they have been used in children with the more severe forms of cerebral palsy. A surgeon implants the drug-delivery pump, which is about the size of a hockey puck, under the skin of the child's abdomen. Then a catheter is threaded—subcutaneously—from the pump to the spinal canal and the pump itself is filled with the medication. The drug, Baclofen, is released in measured doses directly to the facilitated spinal cord network. Because the drug is delivered directly to where it's needed, the spastic circuits at the level of the spinal cord, the dose can be much lower than it would have to be if delivered orally. Baclofen, like Botox, has been found to be a treatment that works well in selected children with quadriplegia.[6]

This treatment is not often used in children with milder forms of spasticity because of the risks of surgery and the need to refill the pump reservoir on a regular basis. However, there has been some relaxation of the pump criteria in recent years. At cerebral palsy meetings, doctors often exchange information informally with one another. At the American Academy of Cerebral Palsy and Development Medicine (AACPDM), the largest of such meetings, I have heard of successful treatment in a toddler with near drowning syndrome, in children with athetoid movement impairments, and most recently in a rapidly growing, heavily muscled male adolescent who was thought to be at risk of progressive body distortion over the next few years. The pump decreased the spastic brain and body habits sufficiently to allow him to grow straight, with no deterioration. I expect there will be more uses for this powerful anti-spasticity treatment in the coming years.

Surgery: Selective Posterior Rhizotomy

A breakthrough neurosurgical treatment of spasticity was brought to the United States by Warwick Peacock, a pediatric neurosurgeon who also did part of his early training in neurosurgery at Toronto's Hospital for Sick Children with Bruce Hendrick.[7] The operation, selective dorsal rhizotomy, is used to decrease spasticity in children with diplegia and hemiplegia by interrupting the spastic reflex arc at the level of the sensory nerves as they enter the spinal cord. Using EMG responses, the surgeon identifies and cuts a proportion of the overactive nerve fibres that carry sensory information from the spastic muscles, interrupting the spastic reflex arc. The negative feedback loop is decreased, and the circuits that control both the spastic and non-spastic antagonist muscles can now work in a more normal fashion with reciprocal activation and inhibition. It only remains to activate the non-spastic antagonist muscles and build strength in both muscle groups.[8]

At first, the response to this surgery was guarded at best. I remember Peacock's first presentation at the AACPDM in the early 1990s. The questions that were asked and the comments that were expressed fell clearly into two camps: a minority like me were excited by the possibilities provided by this surgery, but it was clear from the questions and comments from the audience that the majority were worried about the possible long-term effects of cutting the sensory nerves. Once again, the traditionalists wanted more research.

Nearly twenty years later, there have finally been enough research trials to satisfy at least some of the skeptics that SDR surgery is an effective, proven treatment in children with spastic diplegia.[9] We now know that when done early, progressive body distortion can be avoided. When performed late, that is, when the patients are older, the patients often need orthopedic surgical correction as well. Intensive post-operative muscle strengthening and training the gait into a more normal pattern are required in all cases. Again, this gait retraining is really only effective if done intensively over a period of six to eight weeks or longer.

Orthopedic Surgery: Treating the Body Can Heal the Brain
We have seen that the French investigators "cured" the pseudo-spasticity that occurred in children with brachial plexus injury by turning unbalanced muscle pull into balanced reciprocal muscle pull. What evidence is there that the same improvement can occur in children with cerebral palsy?

Several years ago, I was teaching a course for therapists in the United States. As was my practice, some of the therapists brought in demonstration patients for me to examine. One of them was Chad, an eleven-year-old boy with spastic diplegia affecting both legs. His twin brother did not have CP. His therapist, when she came to the front of the room to introduce him, said that Chad had undergone Single-Event Multilevel Surgery (SEMLS) and was doing really well. She wanted me to examine him and suggest further approaches to therapy now that he was recovering. I wasn't quite sure what to expect.

When I first heard about this surgery, I thought it was just surgeons inventing another heroic, invasive kind of intervention. Some physicians who are not surgeons share something of a prejudice, or at least a vague suspicion that surgeons are prone to charge in and perform complicated and difficult operations just because they can. I say this with affection and admiration, but when I first understood what SEMLS consists of, I was horrified.

The surgery goes on for five or six hours or more. Two surgeons, one on each side of the patient, start at the hip, correcting one deformity after another. This sometimes means moving muscles around, sometimes cutting tendons and lengthening them, and sometimes it's actually breaking bones and turning them into a different position and holding them there with pins. There is no cutting of nerves—they carefully avoid that and focus on correcting the unbalanced muscle and bone biomechanics.[10]

When you consider what they are actually doing, it can make your hair stand on end, and my first reaction on learning about it was decidedly negative. That was my attitude when I first saw Chad.

After telling us about him, the therapist called out his name. He and his brother were standing at the back of the room and they both walked up to join us. They both walked normally. I couldn't tell them apart. As far as their gait was concerned, I could see no difference between them. I stood up and looked for the scars on the boys' legs and that was how I figured out which one had been through the surgery. I examined him and saw that he had a full range of motion. His tone and reflexes were only mildly increased. When I was done, I couldn't understand why he had undergone such a major procedure. In my estimation, he had minimal signs of spastic diplegia. It was hard for me to imagine how a brutal operation like SEMLS could be justified in his case.

Then the therapist showed us the video taken before the surgery.

In a pre-op sequence, Chad was shown walking with a marked crouch gait. He was bent forward at the hips; his back was curved (lordotic) to compensate for tight hip flexor muscles. His knees were bent and he was on his toes. He could walk only a short distance and he had real trouble stopping once he was underway. He didn't walk so much as stagger.

This was a really severe expression of spastic diplegia. He was so affected that a physiotherapist would have been hard put to know where to start. The difference between the staggering boy in the video and the walking boy at the front of the room was astonishing. Chad's body and neurologic function had changed so much because of the surgery that I had little to offer his therapist in the way of recommendations. His walk, when I watched him again, was a bit hesitant. Years of walking with poor balance and a justified fear of falling had had an effect on his confidence. I suggested that he do formal balance training at a higher level. I also thought some martial arts training would be helpful. But overall, the surgeons, Chad, and his therapist had done a superb job of straightening him out, strengthening his weak muscles and pointing him towards a more functional future. The result was spectacular.

Chad made me think again about my attitude towards SEMLS. It also demonstrated that I was not immune from the kind of skepticism that infects us all when we are confronted by something new. We all resist change, even those of us who think of ourselves as revolutionaries.

Probably the most important part of this story is the change in Chad's spasticity or tone. The surgeons had not touched his nerves or treated his brain: they had just rearranged his legs into a proper biomechanical alignment. Yet his spasticity had been significantly reduced. When I understood this—and it took a while—I realized that this is a common finding. I started to ask therapists if they had noted any changes in the level of spasticity after orthopedic surgery. They all agreed that they had. The spastic tone decreases without any direct intervention to the brain, spinal cord, or nerves to the muscles. The orthopedic surgeons had effectively disrupted the negative feedback loop at the level of body alignment. I now think that this is one of the most significant proofs that biomechanical distortions (malalignment) plays a huge part in the progression of spasticity.[11]

It shows what the body can teach the brain.

—— • ——

Every Child Needs a Personal Plan

While there is no global cure for spasticity, there is real hope for serious improvement, especially if a muscle-strengthening regime is incorporated into the therapy selected. We have very effective, evidence-based treatments for established spasticity, such as botulinum toxin and Baclofen pumps, as well as orthopedic and neurosurgery. As we will see in the next chapters, we also have evidence-based protocols of use for earlier treatments with orthotics, for both the upper and lower limbs. We have, as well, evidence-based, intensive training protocols to activate neuroplasticity and teach children new skills.

Whatever the strategy that's adopted, the impaired motor control in the brain (or the nerve in some cases of BPI) is just the starting point. Many brains will improve with time and growth; some will even recover completely. If progressive spasticity is considered a secondary side effect of the interaction between low tone, muscle weakness, and growth, then it can be more effectively treated.

The key problem with cerebral palsy rehabilitation comes down to timing and coordination from multiple practitioners in the medical, surgical, and various therapy professions. Yet these effective treatments are not being offered to patients at the right time, and in the right combination.

Why? It's largely because of the way the CP system works. By the time a child hits age six years, he is surrounded by experts—several therapists, an orthopedic surgeon and/or a neurosurgeon, a CP or BPI developmental expert, a neurologist, a pediatrician, and a wide variety of special education advisers and teachers. Children with more severe problems may also have a speech therapist, an ophthalmologist, and/ or a hearing specialist. Each has their own knowledge base and, more importantly, their own assumptions concerning the child's potential for change. For many of these experts, staying the same is a win.

Although therapists and doctors can be helpful, too often they have low expectations. Most of them don't think that the brain can change and that children with CP can get better. It's partly because most of them see the child with CP for only a few months or a few years. Hardly any of them see the child grow up. When a child is born with brain damage, he's treated by a neonatologist who rarely sees the child after infancy. From birth to age three, the child may go to early intervention or birth-to-three programs, but these last for only three years. Then, from age three to teenage years, the child goes to doctors' and therapists' cerebral palsy clinics, where they are followed closely. Sometime between age four and eight, the orthopedic surgeon is called in to correct deformities in the more severely affected children.

By the time the teenager is entering puberty, most therapy is based in schools. School therapists focus on keeping the child safe and helping him learn, not on improving movement. By then, established common wisdom is that the teen will either stay the same or deteriorate as he grows through puberty. The mildly affected child is expected to, at best, stay the same. At this point, the orthopedic surgeon is generally called in for the second time to correct biomechanical misalignment in the young teenager. Referral to a spasticity management team is highly variable, and generally I have found severe limitations of access for an assessment in the older child or adult.

The system, based on age, creates two problems. First of all, most of the doctors, apart from the pediatrician, see only a part of the natural history of spasticity in cerebral palsy. They don't see how the child with CP grows and develops from birth to teenage years, so it's hard for them to see the development of the spasticity problem, and the real opportunities for prevention and treatment. Second, they do most of the therapy at the wrong time. Most of the standard therapy occurs when the child is age three to puberty. This completely misses the two biggest periods of brain and body growth, when children have a prime opportunity to improve their movement.

We need to do better in treating the motor problems and spasticity that most CP children experience. To give children with cerebral palsy the lives they deserve, we need to change the pediatric rehabilitation system to give patients the appropriate therapy at each stage of their growth and development. In the following chapters, you will meet parents, children, teenagers, and even adults who have found that doing the right thing, at the right time, and in the right order has changed their lives for the better. The revolution is starting from the ground up.

eleven

What to Do in the
First Four Years

With the well-known power of the brain to change and grow, especially in the early years of life, it would be reasonable to assume that babies with an early brain injury would get therapy right away to help them recover from these problems. Sadly, that is often not the case, even though roughly half the children with cerebral palsy can be identified as *at risk* of developing cerebral palsy in the first few months of life.[1] Others will be identified by failure to meet expected milestones over the first year.

Yet the system says that children should wait until problems set in before going to the cerebral palsy clinic. Children with the most severe forms of CP are typically referred to a specialty clinic at age two to three years, but children mildly affected often get no therapy until they are ready for school. They may be seen at a specialty clinic earlier, but they are often judged to be *good enough*, so no intervention, other than intermittent monitoring, is given to them.

This system was set up in the days when doctors thought brains did not change, and that brain injury in babies caused irreversible damage. It was set up at a time when no one expected children with CP to improve very much. And despite the new science of neuroplasticity, which shows that brains can change and heal, this system has not changed since I started in the Follow-Up Clinic at the Hospital for Sick Children over thirty years ago.

It's not right. We are in the midst of a scientific revolution in the care of children with an early neurologic injury. Over the past ten to fifteen years, many innovative therapies that correct maladaptive habits and stimulate neuroplasticity have been tested. Some have demonstrated significant evidence of benefit. Others have had fewer studies completed, but have been found to be promising and, most importantly, safe.[2] These interventions can create real functional change in most children. It's best if the children start therapy as early as possible.

Too often, this does not happen.

Not so long ago, I saw the scope of the problem when I used my blog to conduct an informal survey of parents whose children had been treated in a neonatal intensive care unit and had an early brain injury diagnosed with a brain scan. These children were definitely *at risk* of developing cerebral palsy. I asked my readers what they were told about the nature of the brain injury their child had suffered and what they should do about it. The results were depressing.

Several hundred parents responded, and while there was good news in a few emails, the majority of parents were confused and even angry about the lack of direction and help they were given at discharge. They were told that the future was unknown. I suspect that doctors, hesitant to risk a mistake, are reluctant to say they think it likely that the child will develop cerebral palsy, or even that the child is *at risk* of developing cerebral palsy. So they say, let's wait and see.

Too Little, Too Late

Even when parents are told that there is a high probability of future problems, the bad news is rarely accompanied by a plan of action to give the baby the best possible chance to maximize neuroplasticity and minimize maladaptive habits. I know of no other pediatric disease or disorder where a problem is recognized, in this case an abnormal brain scan, and yet the common wisdom is to sit on our hands and do nothing. Waiting to start treatment until the child is *bad enough* is an outdated, invalid approach.

The first four years are a crucial period in a child's life. It's tragic to waste them by doing nothing. Instead of embarking immediately on therapy, what usually happens is that the child is referred to an early intervention or birth-to-three program. These programs are well intended and most parents report that they are helpful as far as they go. But they don't go nearly far enough for the child with an early neurologic injury. They are designed to gauge the likelihood that a child will have a functional disability. The visiting therapist observes and monitors the infant, usually administering a standardized test to track progress. The first tentative diagnosis is likely to be that the infant is "at risk" of developmental delay. If he is slow in attaining milestones, the "at risk" qualifier is dropped and the diagnosis becomes simply developmental delay.

There are some really big problems with this system. The way the tests are structured means that important problems are missed or ignored. In some areas, a baby with brachial plexus injury that affects only one arm, for example, will not qualify for an early intervention program as the child still scores in the normal range on basic developmental tests. She can perform essential tasks adequately with one undamaged hand and arm. Similarly, for children who may ultimately be given a diagnosis of cerebral palsy, the scoring system tends to downplay maladaptive behaviour if overall function is "good enough" for the child to get by. Poor form is ignored, at least until it becomes "bad enough" to warrant attention as the child grows up. In such cases, the diagnosis of developmental delay ignores the cause and likely evolution of the baby's problems. Specific treatment for CP or BPI is withheld until it is arbitrarily decided to be bad enough for the child to be referred to a clinic for evaluation by an expert.

This is too little, too late.

— • —

The wait-and-see attitude is no longer the standard of care for other early neurologic problems. Autism Speaks and other predominantly parent-led organizations have done an excellent job of bringing the early signs of cognitive/social delay to the awareness of the new parents, professionals, and the general public. In addition to early intervention programs, many in-home treatment programs are now available to help these "at-risk" children. Unfortunately, the parents of a child at risk of motor problems that may evolve into cerebral palsy or the parents of a baby with a definite brachial plexus injury often do not have access to treatment, or the support to get it. Instead they are told to just wait and see.

If the child has had a brain scan in the neonatal period, it is possible to identify the areas of obvious damage and give a realistic assessment of what might be the result. As we have seen, doctors can make an educated assessment of what type of CP is likely. Then diagnosis-specific treatment should be available during the important first four years of exuberant body and brain growth. There is no logical reason to wait. This is the time when there is the best possible chance for normalizing function. Specific best-practice and evidence-informed therapies and treatments are available, but for the most part they are offered only to children whose maladaptive behaviour has become embedded in established neural circuits and, often, has been compounded by issues of tone and body distortion that are difficult to fix. They're offered to the child when she's three or four years old, or later. This makes no sense.

— • —

The first indication of trouble for most children with an early neurologic problem is developmental delay defined as a failure to meet expected milestones on standardized tests of infant behaviour. This is another of those generic terms that cover a wide territory and have little predictive value. There is so much going on in the first four years of the injured child's life. Initially, the brain may be in a state of shock. At best, recovery is slow—it takes time. But when recovery begins, all the extraordinary changes that transform the helpless infant into a curious and energetic toddler kick in. The brain grows and, as it grows, the part that was damaged stays the same size. The damaged sector is a big part of the brain initially, but as the brain grows, the damaged bit becomes proportionately smaller. It is obvious that the child's potential for functional recovery increases with time.

Brain growth has other implications. The infant is becoming aware of his own body. He begins to explore the world. Various functions like speech and language comprehension come online. If you graph maximum brain neuroplasticity from birth through to age eight, it is high at birth and then slows and levels off at four to six years. This level of growth is still higher than it is in an adult brain, though, and it stays this way until the preteen enters puberty. Then comes another four- to six-year burst of growth. Both the early (up to age four to six) and later teenage years are peak periods of neuroplasticity. Unfortunately, most rehabilitation therapy is given to children between four and twelve years of age, when there is less potential for the brain to change and heal than in the earlier years. Standard therapy for cerebral palsy also misses both the early and late periods of peak body growth when the child is most at risk of developing progressive spasticity and body distortion.

Stimulating Baby Brain Neuroplasticity

The baby brain, while still immature, is capable of far more than we have traditionally supposed. Babies are curious and responsive to novel stimuli. Studies have suggested how this information can be put to practical use. However counterintuitive it may seem, it may make sense to dispense with the baby talk parents sometimes use with their baby. Although the child with a brain injury typically takes longer than other children to learn how to react to words, some studies suggest it's better to talk to a baby as you would an adult. Anne Fernald, the author of one such study, wrote, "You're building intelligence through language. It's making networks of meaning that will then help the child learn new words."[3] Baby brains love novelty. Think of this from the baby's perspective. If adults who talk baby talk all day surround them, how can their brains learn and develop the associative networks that are the basis of language? Raised expectations lead to an elevated outcome—and not just when it comes to learning language skills.

Research suggests other strategies for stimulating a baby or toddler's development. Hearing and vision are two of the earliest-developing brain skills. A significant number of full-term babies with asphyxia (low oxygen) at birth have damage to the part of their brains that processes visual signals. It is called cortical visual impairment (CVI). These babies have diminished control over their eye movements: they wander all over in a random manner, a condition specialists call roving nystagmus. Early in my training, I was taught that this type of nystagmus meant that the child would be blind, not from an eye problem, but from brain damage to the occipital lobes of the brain. It was considered a permanent problem. But, like so many other firm diagnoses of the past, this too has turned out to be incorrect. I have personally seen many infants with CVI whose parents sought out early help from an optometrist trained in remedial eye exercises.[4] In many, the nystagmus disappears over the first years of life. The children may still have some problems, like a lazy eye, but they are not blind. I now think that our earlier practice of "wait and see" what would happen with the eyes led to a development of non-use in the visual areas of the brain. Use it or lose it seems to be a universal principle in human bodies and brains. Again, rather than waiting until the child is two, three, or four years old, we should be initiating therapies that take advantage of the young brain's capacity to change.

Stretching and Massage

The same potential for improvement exists for the baby's developing motor system. Babies with an injured brain start out floppy and weak, and as they grow, we know that 80 percent of the ones who will go on to be diagnosed with cerebral palsy start to tighten up, developing the motor signs of spasticity. Every athlete knows that tight muscles respond to massage and stretching, and it seems reasonable that some harmless yet effective treatments could be started earlier. It is common practice to recommend massage and stretching once CP is diagnosed, but research studies done later in childhood when spasticity is firmly established have demonstrated that stretching did not have much effect on established spasticity.[5]

Why not try it earlier? Rather than jump to the conclusion that tissue management doesn't work, I think it is a more reasonable plan to start this treatment earlier. Starting at four years or later is clearly too late.

Several research studies have shown that an infant can benefit from massage and stretching. There are established protocols and even classes to teach parents how to do it properly. When premature babies, still in the NICU, are massaged, measureable improvements have been documented.[6]

Most parents know this. Before the child leaves the hospital, they are almost always shown some basic movements to practise with their baby. In my experience, however, they rarely do it as often as it should be done. A peak-performance athlete in training stretches many times a day and never when the muscles are cold. Athletes stretch after a warm-up exercise or after a warm shower or bath. They might apply a heating pad to troublesome muscle groups to deal with localized tightness. All these are techniques that can also be used for the infant at risk of developing cerebral palsy. One smart mother taught me about whole-bed heating pads, commonly used by massage therapists to keep their clients warm during a treatment. She put one in her two-year-old son's bed and turned it on for ten to fifteen minutes in the morning before helping him out of bed. She found it far easier to stretch him after this warm-up.

Experienced athletes understand that stretching and massage improve recovery, as well as maintaining flexibility. Most adults automatically stretch when they have been hunched over a computer for a long time. My dog stretches every time she gets up from a nap. Babies stretch in the same way when they wake up. Children who have an early neurologic injury can't do it on their own. They need help. It seems obvious to me that we should be doing this work with them.

In my opinion, tissue management with massage and proper stretching should be part of the daily routine of all children with any form of early muscle imbalance that limits their ability to stretch independently. At least twice a day, every day, until they stop growing.

Start Right, Stay Straight

Babies first investigate their hands with their mouth, and then gradually, between three and six months, they use them to reach for things that they see. Even at the stage of independent sitting, those wiggly bits at the end of his arms can fascinate a baby. Babies with an early brain or nerve injury rarely go through this early exploratory stage. They start off in the newborn period with a problem of weakness or low tone, called hypotonia. This makes it hard for the baby to bring the hand to the mouth. Parents can help by supporting the infant's arm and hand in position. The goal is to keep the hands first in the mouth for exploration and later in the visual field. Babies with low vision can still mouth their hands, and if you add a bell to a brightly coloured wristband, they will develop a sense of their hands in space.

If they are not supported in this early stage, they will still try to find their hand, but at a cost. When the child with impaired motor control tries to get her hand up to her mouth, she turns on all the muscles, causing the hand to fist, the elbow to flex, and the shoulder to lift up. This sets off a chain reaction that stiffens the same side of the body. The medical term for this whole-body reaction is "activity-dependent tone." The brain is sending signals to the body, but they are a generalized call to action and lack normal isolated control. This overreaction by a damaged nervous system is the first sign of developing spasticity.

Once the infant can be put in the upright position, trunk support is the first requirement. Floppy, weak babies cannot support their trunk on their own and further development of arm control depends upon a stable trunk. Experienced therapists, particularly those trained in the Bobath neurodevelopmental approach, know how to quickly facilitate a normal sitting position by supporting the baby with their hands. Unfortunately, the therapist's hands do not go home with the parents.

I was first introduced to a range of compressive garments by pediatric occupational therapist Kim Barthel. She showed me that firm compressive garments seemed to calm children on the autism spectrum and those with other sensorimotor problems. In the cerebral palsy world, there are several different supportive garments in use that have been designed to provide external support for weak muscles. It took me years to realize that these garments do not just support the trunk; they also improve proprioceptive awareness. They give the child a better sense of where he is in space.

It's a case of everybody knowing something without consciously knowing it. All therapists know that when a child is trying to perform a new activity, they hold on to them firmly and put them in the right position. Generally they think of this as providing support, which it is, but they are also giving them body awareness. Try this: stand up, lift your arms out to the side at about shoulder height, and then shut your eyes. All the little muscles in your feet will start going crazy. Some people have difficulty balancing in this position. Now open your eyes. Lift your arms to the side again, shut your eyes, and lift one foot off the ground. When you shut your eyes, you take away your visuomotor feedback and you have to depend on your body to know where it is. Unless you do yoga or train your balance reactions regularly, you will be shocked by your lack of body awareness. In most children with cerebral palsy, proprioceptive awareness is poorly developed.

I am often asked if compressive support garments lead to muscle weakness. The exact opposite is true! These garments allow the child to strengthen her trunk muscles in the correct position. If the child sits slumped forward, all the trunk muscles are out of alignment. The muscles of the back are in a stretched, elongated position and the belly muscles are shortened. This is important because every muscle of our body has its own optimum length. In a shorter or longer position, the amount of force the muscle can produce is limited.

Therapists know how to limit activity-dependent tone with positioning and support from the hands. The use of compressive support garments is a complementary technique: the therapist can demonstrate improvement with proper handling; the vest allows the parent to "take the therapist's hands home."

Correct alignment leads to awareness, which is just as necessary in the toddler and young child as it is in the infant. If the hand is not in view, the brain will forget about it. If the hand is not supported in a position of use, the child will not use it. Once the child knows about the hand, the child can use it to develop new skills. This concept is not complicated: the brain pays attention to what it is aware of, so the most important task is to facilitate awareness in the best possible alignment.

All these interventions are intended to prevent the development of maladaptive habits that, if they are allowed to develop, require different kinds of intervention.

— • —

There are two facts to keep in mind about children with CP. They all have some degree of impaired balance. What's more, the first sign of increased spasticity in the legs is over-active extensor muscles. These are the strongest muscles that respond first to the impaired signals from a damaged brain. The extensor tone in the legs tends to put children up on their toes and push them into a falling-forward position. This makes their balance even worse. Both children and adults find it difficult to balance without a stable base. Think of the able-bodied child learning to stand and walk. The first few times he gets up, he promptly falls down again. And again. And again. The child with CP has to learn by the same hard process that is made infinitely more complicated by being up on his toes.

Treatments that maintain alignment *allow* more normal movement and growth. Up on their toes is hard for children with CP, but if their feet are supported in a normal position, they can better learn *how to do* a skill. Again, a key difference between an adult with a stroke and a child with hemiplegia is the child has a growing body and *any* tone change will distort growth. None of the *how-to* therapies will work as intended (or at all) if we have allowed the body to become distorted. Proper alignment is a precondition of good form.

Solene was born with a malformation on one side of her brain that caused a severe seizure disorder. She had a hemispherectomy at three months of age. Solene's parents have been working on giving their daughter the support she needs to stand and walk. I insisted they get braces for Solene's feet to support her. Form, I explained to the parents, matters a lot. We had to stop Solene from acquiring bad walking habits. It was more important for her to learn to walk properly, correctly, than to learn to walk any which way.

"We had not heard this before," Solene's parents told me. "We heard the opposite. A lot of people were pushing function. They said, just get her up. Get her doing this and get her doing that."

That wasn't my view: repeating bad movements is just building pathways into the brain to have bad movement. Learning to walk badly just teaches the toddler to do bad better. These children have impaired motor control to start and will not spontaneously correct maladaptive patterns.

They just perfect them, wiring the abnormal pattern into their brains, and in the process, they set up the progressive negative feedback loop we call spasticity.

———— • ————

Parents of small children with the early signs of cerebral palsy commonly ask me, "Will he walk?" followed quickly by, "When?" I think this is an incorrect focus for a child with an early neurologic problem. Ninety-nine percent of children with hemiplegia end up walking and up to 98 percent of children with diplegia also walk with or without aids. In children with quadriplegia, walking takes longer and they may need more interventions. By definition, all the children with Level I to III cerebral palsy, or mild to moderate severity, will walk either independently (60 percent) or with assistance from crutches or a cane.[7]

Most people with CP, then, will walk. The real question is what kind of walking will they do? If they are pushed to walk, and if we accept bad form when they do walk, we are setting them up for significant long-term problems. The maladaptive habit will become established. As they grow, increasing spasticity and biomechanical distortion will be the inevitable result. This body distortion leads to chronic musculoskeletal pain in over half of adults with cerebral palsy.

As they grow and mature, children want to move and they should move but within the limits that prevent harm to their growing bodies. Having a child wait to walk until he can do it well brings up a conflict with current thinking about stimulating neuroplasticity. Children learn by experience and movement is a necessary part of learning. Movement teaches awareness of spatial relationships and is a necessary part of learning to socialize with other children. Happily, there are some innovative ways to teach young children to acquire these skills before they are able to manage walking about independently.

Dr. Cole Galloway from the University of Delaware has created Go Baby Go cars for infants as young as six months to give them movement experiences.[8] These inexpensive cars are modified children's "ride on" toys and can be produced for a very low cost, compared to the thousands of dollars for a powered wheelchair. The lack of commercially available power wheelchairs for children under the age of three years started his initial search for an affordable alternative. The toy cars are modified with switches and body supports, individualized for each child's need. For example, a child with a persistent head-down position will have a car acceleration switch that is activated only when she lifts her head and presses back on the switch. A more advanced model for a child walking with crutches would be rigged so that the car can move forward only when the child is standing tall, with his feet properly supported, actively strengthening his legs. Yet another has the child doing sit-to-stand and stand-to-sit movements to propel the car. This is a brilliant concept that allows the child with a physical limitation to play with his peers while actually improving his odds of one day walking unaided with good form.

"Practice Does Not Make Perfect. Only Perfect Practice Makes Perfect."
—Vince Lombardi

After good body alignment is achieved, the child must practise, practise, practise. We know that abnormal movement patterns develop as the child tries to move against gravity. This is easily demonstrated. The infant may have perfectly normal four-point movements lying on her back on the floor but have increased tone as soon as she is first put into a sitting or standing position. The arms and hands tighten up automatically as she tries to balance to protect herself from falling. This is the early stage of spasticity. Skilled therapists can show parents how to minimize this tone with handling techniques, but this alone may not be enough. For one thing, you can't take the therapist's skilled hands home with you. For another, one or two hours a week in therapy is useless as a sole intervention. No athlete has learned a sport, no musician has learned to play an instrument, and no dancer has mastered a difficult routine without a whole lot of practice. A toddler needs that kind of practice too.

The best therapists find ways to use the out-of-gravity principle, combined with their knowledge of neuroplasticity, to develop techniques that successfully prevent or replace maladaptive habits. Suzanne Davis Bombria makes good use of a device developed in Europe, the Universal Exercise Unit.

"If I am working on walking and I see a pattern that I don't like, I am not just going to work on walking. I am going to come up with new ways to have that body move," Suzanne explains. "For example, I have been working with a child who has one side of her body that rotates in and the knee collapses. I am doing climbing with her. I get her to climb a wall to change her walking habit.... I have a cage—it's actually called the Universal Exercise Unit.... I am first and foremost an NDT therapist, but I will use any tool, anybody's toolbox that works.

"The cage looks like the wire material that is used in closets, the white shelving wire. It is a six-by-six-foot cube that has one side open. It has walls and a roof. I can set the child up in bungee cords and have them move around. I can add pulleys and weights so they are strengthening.... The climbing [in the cage] is something she enjoys. It is an activity that is fun and it is part of play. That is part of neuroplasticity too, and neuromotor learning. She sees it as play and it is like any kid going to a playground, park, or climbing wall. She is having a grand time doing it, but it is exercise therapy and she feels that, and she wants to keep challenging herself to do it.

"[Sometimes] I would take bungee cords and attach them to my cage at a height that is like parallel bars; only it is giving her a lot less support than parallel bars. It is only a bungee cord and it is very dynamic, so it challenges her to put the work back into her legs and learn balance. It might be similar to walking in the water. If a child is unsteady, just walking along, gravity happens and you are gone. But in the cage with bungee cord support, when you are walking, it slows down your fall. You have the chance to correct yourself without your therapist catching you.

"We did a lot of standing with the bungees. We were teaching her to walk. We did it in tiny, tiny little steps because I always think I have to break things down to small milli-metres ... our kids have to have it so broken down. For her, I went from a place where I could hold her hands and she would take some steps, to a point where I am holding a little dolly and she is going to hold the other end of the dolly. It becomes more dynamic. And then we used a little bungee cord and she could hug the bungee cord. And then I just held on to one end of the bungee and she held on to the other end. And then one day my husband came home with a helium balloon. I had been looking for that next step, I needed some-thing else. When he came home with the balloon with a little weight at the end of it and I said, Oh, my gosh! This was my answer. He gave her the balloon and she walked with that.

"She is an independent walker now. She walks up and down steps. It is amazing, her recovery."

As Suzanne says, children need incredible amounts of practice, and making it fun and challenging is an absolute requirement. Great therapists find ways to challenge their patients to do more, just as a great coach or tennis pro starts with where you are and figures out the next small steps to take you to the next level.

Another technique that I've mentioned previously is water exercise. I know of no other form of therapy that is better for all-around strengthening and improving cardiovascular fitness in children and adults with a neurologic problem. Tone increases as the child moves against gravity and it decreases when he is in a gravity-reduced environment. For toddlers and young children, water is a fun-filled play environment where they can escape from the negative pull of gravity.

Just about any flotation device that holds the child's body upright will work in the young. Traditional life jackets do not work as they tend to keep the child at a backwards angle to keep the face out of the water. The idea is just to support children upright in the water and then encourage them to move. It will take a bit of time, but it is a novel challenge and they will eventually discover how to activate all their muscles and to fire them reciprocally. On land, in gravity, the bully, spastic muscles dominate, but in the water the muscles quickly learn to relax and work cooperatively. I have seen great results, even in children with complex forms of cerebral palsy like athetoid quadriplegia, a movement disorder that affects balance and control of all four limbs. I tried water exercise—really water play—with one young girl who was so limited that at nearly five years of age, she could not sit independently, let alone stand or walk. This is what her mother said about a summer water exercise program: "The most amazing thing that came out of the water program was independence for my daughter. She is so physically limited, that before the summer, she was never without an adult to hold or support her. Now, in the water she had unrestricted movement. She could swim on her own. We could swim together as a family for fitness or fun. It was the perfect way to enjoy the hot summer weather. She began to wake up every morning asking to go swimming or saying that she had a wonderful dream that she swam to one place or another with one of her friends. I will never forget the look on her face the first time she jogged from one end of the pool to the other on her own."

— • —

In the early years we have to use our imagination to think of ways to stimulate the young brain to develop as normally as possible. The take-away lessons about neuroplasticity are simple:

1. The brain learns from the body, so you have to start out life moving in the right way. We have to provide the needed supports so that the child learns to move well from the start.

2. Once a maladaptive brain or body habit is established, it is hard to replace with a better movement pattern.

   Habits are hard to change, so you have to give the brain something new to do.

   The way to work *out of habit* is to present the brain with a novel, challenging task and then let the child's brain figure out how to accomplish it. We learn by experience, and if we can make that learning fun, it is easier to get the necessary practice.

3. Early walking can result in bad walking. Once the child is given an *at-risk* of cerebral palsy diagnosis, a common reaction is to spend all the parents' time and effort on movement skills. This is a mistake. We have to give the baby brain time to heal and time

to mature. Pushing early walking most commonly results in learning to walk badly.

4. Function follows form. Any therapist or program that advises parents against using biomechanical supports that are needed to produce good alignment is arguing against all that we know about human biomechanics. Even peak-performance athletes, with near-perfect neuromotor systems, wear supportive garments and use orthotics to help their bodies maintain good form.

5. Cut out the baby talk. The speaking, hearing, thinking parts of the baby brain need stimulation too. Speaking to a young child in adult language can help his brain develop.

It is time for a change from a *wait-and-see* paradigm to one including active interventions to *maximize neuroplasticity and minimize maladaptive habits* in the early years of life. Thankfully, even if the child missed these active interventions in the first four years, neuroplasticity and the possibility of higher functional gains is lifelong for the vast majority of children and adults.

twelve

What to Do in the Middle Years

By the time a child is referred to a cerebral palsy or brachial plexus centre for therapy, he has a well established movement pattern. The negative feedback loop is in place with wired-in circuits in the brain and well-practised maladaptive movement habits in the body. By then, the chance to prevent problems has vanished. We're now dealing with established habits of the mind and body, and potentially the body distortions that accompany it.

Yet as we will see, there are proven therapies and treatments, including surgery, that can help children learn new habits of walking and moving. However, this exciting news of real hope has apparently not made it to the front lines of care. Iona Novak, one of the acknowledged leaders in evidence-based and best-practice intervention for children with cerebral palsy, paints a depressing picture:

Outdated care is regrettably being provided to children with cerebral palsy. Consistent with other fields (of medicine) 10% to 40% are not offered proven effective interventions, and another 20% receive harmful or ineffective interventions. Furthermore, the persistent preference for conservative late diagnosis of cerebral palsy following failed milestones conflicts with current neuroscience evidence. Very early intervention, close to the time of injury, is now advised to optimize neuroplasticity.[1]

In other words, the standard therapies, now outdated, fail to take full advantage of neuroplasticity and to mitigate the adverse effects of growth.

No parent should accept that her child with CP cannot get better after age six. And as it turns out, many don't. I have gradually come to the realization that the greatest advocates for these young patients are their parents. Parents can deal first with the pediatrician, who is often the one physician who sees the child and family most consistently over the years and can coordinate the management of complex problems in the home.

If parents are directing the care for their children, it's important to set age-dependent goals for the child, especially when they're contending with children past the first few years of maximal neuroplasticity. Changing or replacing maladaptive habits in these children is hard work. The key to change is to focus on doing the right thing(s), at the right time, and in the right order. The age and stage of brain development is the starting point.

In a child older than three to four years, we assume any spontaneous recovery from the initial injury is completed. If the child has well-established maladaptive habits, the first challenge is see how much his brain has recovered. Step one is to reveal this recovery. We know children with CP walk with the established pattern of their particular type of cerebral palsy: hemiplegia, diplegia, quadriplegia, or the less common mixed forms of cerebral palsy. That is their *usual* pattern and it both informs us about the likelihood of co-morbidities and allows us to monitor for typical patterns of body distortion. This is a good thing, but it does not inform us of the degree of brain recovery. For this information you have to look at their running skills and other higher-order abilities. What is their best performance? If they run well, the corticospinal system is in good enough shape to allow real improvement. If the child with hand involvement can catch a ball with both hands in play, her brain is capable of improved function. The key point is the habits, representing *usual* performance, are the default mode in the brain. You only see, and only can work with, recovered brain when you do novel, challenging tasks.

By looking at the best performance, we now know the potential, what they are able to do at this age. The next task is to get them to use their best performance more consistently. As I have written before, even athletes stop to correct malalignment issues before they try to improve performance. The same body rules apply to the child with an established cerebral palsy movement pattern.

Step two is making sure the child has the best possible functional alignment. As I explained in an earlier chapter, function follows form. It's a universal principle of how bodies work. What they learn now depends upon what they do. If they are walking with poor form, practising the same thing will not make them walk properly. They will only learn to walk badly better. If the older child has a hand that is persistently fisted, that hand is not much use to the child and it will be ignored. Alignment is vital.

Upper-Limb Alignment

One of my favourite research trials used a simple experimental design that tested the hand function of a group of four- to eight-year-olds with hemiplegia. Each child had a baseline test that measured just how often the hand on the side of the hemiplegia was used as an assist in tasks such as holding a paper while the other hand cut it with scissors. Called the Assisting Hand Assessment, or AHA, this is a well-standardized test with good reproducibility. After the initial test of their hand function, the children were sent home and told to return for retesting the next week. For the second test, each child was fitted with a brightly coloured hand splint that kept his wrist in a good functional position and supported the thumb in a normal position.

Immediately after the second test, the hand splint was removed and the child sent home without it for another week. Test number three was done without the splint on after a further week.

The results were astonishing. With the hand splint on, there was an extremely significant improvement measured by the AHA test. The chance of the improvement occurring by chance was less than one in a thousand. Additionally, there was no difference between the first and third tests, both done without the hand splint. This result proved that the improvement seen on the middle test could not be attributed to the children learning the test.[2]

A simple splint improved function immediately. Yet the sad truth is that most therapists do not prescribe them and parents, even when they have been given a splint, rarely use them. Over the years, I have repeatedly asked, *Why not?*

The change is immediate and the function is improved.

If the wrist and hand are in good alignment, the child is better able to use the hand, and if she uses it, we now know that those atrophied, disused parts of her brain have a chance to wake up and be useful. But, without use, there can be no persistent change.

In the early 1980s, Edward Taub proved that Constraint Induced Movement Therapy could teach an adult with a stroke to use the affected hand once again. This approach to treatment was initially resisted in pediatric neurorehabilitation, but there are now over twenty randomized controlled trials that confirm its worth in the rehabilitation of the upper limb in children with cerebral palsy.[3] Children with hemiplegia can learn, in a two- to four-week intensive program, how to use their spastic hand in a more useful fashion. There is no logical reason to think that CIMT will not work equally well in children with a brachial plexus injury with recovered nerve function.

Functional brain scans in children with cerebral palsy before and after CIMT training camps have demonstrated actual changes in their brain activity that correspond to their improved skills.[4] CIMT in adults with learned non-use and children with developmental non-use have both benefited from this treatment.

Another intervention, Hand–Arm Bilateral Intensive Therapy (HABIT), has been studied as a solo intervention and with CIMT. HABIT does not constrain the child's more functional hand, but rather the intensive training program is filled with tasks that encourage the child to use both hands together, for example, catching a large ball; has been proven safe and effective; and has resulted in measurable brain improvement.[5]

This all is good news on the surface. Relatively inexpensive wrist and hand splints can provide good alignment in a child with a good range of motion in the joints. If the spasticity habit is too well established, medications like Botox injections can tone down the tight muscles and serial applications of casts can restore normal joint movement in most cases. In the best of all possible worlds, the child would be able to have the specific interventions that he needs (the right thing) added to the treatment program sequentially (in the right order). It is also important to recognize that when parents and therapists move heaven and earth to arrange the time to do an intensive period of CIMT or HABIT, many children start off without the best preparation. The hand alignment should be corrected before the intensive program that will train them *how to do* new skills.

Gait Training

Proven effective interventions for improving hand function are relatively recent additions to the therapy toolbox, but therapists have been trying to teach children how to walk for years and years. Unfortunately, most of the focus for many has been teaching the child *how to* walk first without taking care of alignment issues. As I have said elsewhere, untreated spasticity inevitably leads to body distortion and chronic pain.

If the child is given adequate bracing early, the tone in the legs can be dramatically reduced. The most commonly used lower-limb brace is the ankle foot orthotic. Unfortunately, a survey by the American Orthotic and Prosthetic Association discovered that the average age for this brace to be prescribed was three to four years. At this age, in most children with cerebral palsy, the ship has sailed. They have established spasticity and forcing the foot into a rigid brace does not work. Countless parents will attest to the experience of ill-fitting braces that are not only uncomfortable but cause bruising and painful blisters. Most parents stop using them. And the negative feedback loop progresses unchecked.

The problem here is doing the right thing at the wrong time. Using AFOs early gives the still supple foot support in the correct alignment and inhibits the spastic reflex loop. But they have to be used consistently, whenever the child is upright, to have this effect. In most cases, with established spasticity, the child will need to have one or more of the effective treatments for spasticity *to allow* more normal movement before any type of leg brace is likely to work.

Treating spasticity and correcting alignment are the primary requirements. In children with severe spastic diplegia, affecting both legs, neurosurgeons are interrupting the negative feedback loop with SDR surgery as early as in two-year-olds. Botox and other forms of botulinum toxin are FDA approved at two years as well. Additionally, some innovative orthopedic surgeons have developed relatively non-invasive surgical procedures to help correct alignment in the early years. Selective Percutaneous Myofascial Lengthening, also known as SPML or PERCS, is a day-surgery procedure that has been shown to help interrupt the progression of muscle and tendon tightness in the leg.

In Chapter 10 I reviewed some of the presently available options for correcting established spasticity and restoring alignment. Most children with cerebral palsy will need to have several of these interventions. In my experience, they should be used earlier. Once the muscle tightness is decreased and the alignment of the bones and joints restored, the work of making new positive movement habits is next.

Replacing Habits

Replacing habits with new ones at any age is hard work and requires focus on one goal at a time. This is how humans learn. Athletes and coaches know the *one at a time* rule—a B-class tennis player does not work on everything that is wrong about his technique at once. It is a gradual pro-cess of relearning and building skills one on another. Even peak-performance athletes, with exceptional motor skills, cannot work on more than one thing at a time. To succeed, the children need what top athletes have—a coach.

I have used an athletic approach to the treatment of CP for years, and I've found it helps. There is a real overlap between coaching athletes and coaching children with cerebral palsy or brachial plexus injury. In fact, I like to think I treat the children like the athletes they really are. To start with, whether you're a world-class athlete or a seven-year-old girl with CP, you need a goal—like walking independently. Then you need to break it into a series of short-term goals. The short-term goals should be *measurable* so that everyone can see the progress and update the programs as necessary. All the therapists involved in the care of the child should be working towards the same goals.

Goal-oriented therapy made perfect sense to the mother of a seven-year-old girl I once treated. She's an engineer, and in her field, goal-oriented projects are essential: "If you are creating a solution to a problem such as redoing or streamlining a process in a factory, you need to have measurable metrics to see the effects of the intervention you are proposing. It should be the same with therapy. If you target a certain area or propose the use of a certain set of exercises, you need to measure the progress to know where to move forward and to assess when you are ready to change.

"With the help of Karen, we got focused and took control of the therapy program, working on measurable goals that were a priority for us and having all our therapists work together to create a plan for our daughter."

With clear, measurable goals, we could see the little girl improve almost immediately. She gained strength and abilities right away. Yet not everyone involved in her care was initially on board. "This was a big change from how they had been doing things," her mother says. "It involves a time commitment from our therapists and us. We need to do the home program we are given, take videos, and report on our progress. Our therapists have to plan ahead of our therapy sessions and continuously review and update our program and our short-term goals. It was and continues to be a challenge to get our therapists to communicate effectively, but it's worth the effort."

All the research in cerebral palsy supports the concept that targeted, intermittent, intensive training gives the best chance of improving the level of performance. Think of the change in performance achieved at a hockey, golf, or tennis camp. One, two, or a few weeks of focused intensive work on a goal that is important to a person creates change. And with change comes motivation. People will try harder to reach an objective when they see positive results.

There are many techniques that have been proven to help children with CP learn to cast off their bad habits and reach their full potential for better movement. Water exercise with a Wet Vest, for instance, allows children to integrate and actively participate with able-bodied peers without damaging their bodies.

Jimmy arrived at the Magee Clinic from the United States for assessment when he was eight years old. He had Level III cerebral palsy and used forearm crutches to get around. He was a slightly built child, and his problem seemed to be as much about muscle weakness as it was about spasticity, which seemed quite mild. I worked out a plan for him to do some intensive water work over the summer. He normally spent most of the summer in the family's backyard pool with his two older brothers. He didn't swim but bounced around in a standard life jacket. When he first tried the Wet Vest, within a few days, he was able to jog about the pool with ease. His strength and endurance increased from the beginning, when he could jog for ten minutes at a time, to the point where he was racing around the pool all day. His parents sent me an email the day he beat both brothers in racing the length of the pool.

When he left school in June, his therapists warned his parents that he might need to use a wheelchair for safety and mobility when in a few years he would move to a larger middle school. After a summer of intensive practice in the pool, that option was taken off the table. When he returned to school in the fall, he was walking independently for longer distances; he was able to manage moving about the classroom and could even safely go up and down the stairs between classrooms.

In the young child, this type of change is not magical. It just requires figuring out what is impeding progress. Jimmy did not need more therapy to teach him how to walk. His biggest problem was muscle weakness and poor cardiovascular fitness. Jimmy was tired all the time. He wasn't exercising as would be usual for a child his age. He never would have cooperated with a program of two to four hours a day of resistive muscle strengthening, but playing in the water was a novel challenge out of gravity. All that time spent jogging in the water strengthened his body and lungs, but it also taught his brain how to initiate a more normal pattern of reciprocal movement in his legs. That is why it worked so well to improve his walking. He only cared that it was fun and he beat his brothers in a race.

Hippotherapy, riding a horse, is another good example of child-active rehabilitation that is a promising intervention.[6] In the push for full integration of the special needs child, it is also important to recognize the role of adapted sports programs like BlazeSports or AccesSportAmerica[7] that challenge the child to achieve new goals in social integration and improved fitness and health. Novel, challenging tasks spark neuroplasticity.

It is clearly time for a change in the established routines of neurorehabilitation in children. Eighty percent of children with CP have a mild to moderate level of impairment. With all the medical, surgical, and, most importantly, therapy interventions developed in the past two decades, every one of these children can reasonably expect to improve their function. In the old days, before we knew what we do now about human neuroplasticity, there was not much we could do about the motor problems of children with CP. But now we know what needs to be done, and how to do it. Waiting to intervene until the child is *bad enough* is untenable in the twenty-first century.

thirteen

How Teens Can Make New Habits

The teenage years are especially difficult for children with cerebral palsy. One long-term study that tracked children with CP from age two to twenty-one showed that when the children hit puberty, the ones with the least impairment stayed the same in terms of motor function, while those with more serious impairment (Level III, IV, and V) actually got worse. All the children enrolled in the study were born between 1986 and 1996 and were seen in several regional CP centres in Ontario.

This study may be depressing for parents, but it provides valuable information about the development of children with CP until they become adults.

The researchers repeatedly tested children with a well-standardized assessment of gross and fine motor function.[1] On the basis of these results, each child was assigned to one of five levels using the GMFCS. At yearly intervals thereafter, they were reassessed to see if there was any change in their functional level.

All the children showed some initial improvement in their function in the first years of life. The most seriously affected children improved up to age three and four, while the least impaired showed improvement up to age seven to eight. Then they stayed the same for several years, which happened to be the very years when children with CP were in standard therapy.

When the children reached puberty, the study showed, the story took a nasty turn. The children with the most serious level of impairment (Level III, IV, and V) declined in terms of their motor function. The less-impaired children stayed the same.

What does this study show? You might think it simply shows what will happen to children with different levels of CP. That's how the traditional thinking goes: once a child's GMFCS level is determined between age three and eight, the CP establishment figures that the level of function in a child will stay the same or get worse. After all, in their view, cerebral palsy is a *permanent* disorder of movement and posture.

I disagree. I believe this result documents widespread treatment failure.

We now know that the child's brain keeps maturing and developing new abilities throughout childhood and adolescence. So, once again, we are faced with a big anomaly. By the teenage years, the initial, one-time brain injury has healed, to whatever extent that it can. The remaining normal brain continues to grow and mature in function. Logically, the child's function should continue to improve.

So what's happening? Why do children with CP decline or stay the same during their teenage years, just when their brains are growing and developing at an extraordinary rate?

First, the overall expectation for change is low. As the old coaching adage puts it, "If you set your standards low enough, it is easy to be satisfied with your performance."

Second, the GMFCS measures *"usual performance rather than what they are known to be able to do at their best."*[2] This is misleading. It is now clear that every motor function in a child with cerebral palsy has a range from best to worst performance. A child with an abnormal walking pattern might score at a Level I or II, but the test does not consider the ability to run, jump, pivot, and kick a soccer ball even better than other boys with no CP. Those *above normal* skills don't count for the test, so he's still scored at Level I or II. It is his *usual performance*. In other words, the test measures the lowest skill level, the habits, which do not change with the standard treatment methods available at the turn of the century.

Third, children chosen for the study received the standard treatments that prevailed in the 1990s, before neuroplasticity changed the game. They did not have the benefit of modern spasticity management! "Children were excluded [*from the study*]," the authors explained, "if they had a selective dorsal rhizotomy, had received botulinum toxin injections in the lower limbs for spasticity management or were receiving intrathecal baclofen."[3] In other words, the children in the study were not getting the twenty-first-century treatments that we now know work. They only got the standard treatment that prevailed in the 1990s.

It's no surprise that the seriously affected teens in this study deteriorated when they didn't get the benefit of modern spasticity management to stop problems like progressive spasticity as they grew through puberty. We now know that unchecked spastic habits lead to inevitable functional deterioration, and the complicated orthopedic management that is required is still not widely available. Yet the data in this study are used to predict a child's potential for improvement over time, and advise on treatments. The authors even go so far as to use out-of-date data to advise parents on surgical interventions. "From these data we can see that, for example, it would not be appropriate to perform extensive gait correction surgery on a child in level IV when their prognosis for motor function is for transfer and, at best, limited walking with primarily wheelchair use for mobility."[4]

This is not true: if children at Level IV have the benefit of current treatments both for spasticity management and orthopedic correction, some will improve their level of function.[5]

The Teenage Brain

Teenagers gain up to 40 percent more brainpower during puberty. The teen years are the second peak period of neuroplasticity. There is not much change in the size of the brain at this point. Most of the change is in maturation of functions and improvements of the interconnections between different brain areas. At the same time of these major changes in the brain, the preteen enters the last major body growth spurt with the onset of puberty.

A teenager in puberty is like a peak-performance athlete on steroids. Teenagers are growing rapidly because they have excess amounts of growth hormones, anabolic steroids, and sex hormones flooding the system. Puberty is a prime time for both the brain and body to grow, and it happens sooner than you may think. The average girl in North America begins puberty at age eleven (with a range from eight to fourteen); boys typically begin puberty at twelve (with a range from nine to fourteen or even older). Typically, it takes girls two to four years to fully mature, while boys usually take four to six years. During this time, their brains are maturing and developing connections. Most importantly, their frontal lobes, the centres of higher cognitive function, are coming online. This means is that teenagers start to develop their own opinions and can be motivated to work hard for a distant goal. They now can access new parts of the brain to improve both motor functions and speech.

As their prefrontal cortex matures, teens are capable of abstract thought, planning, and decision making. A motivated teenager is now able to do focused training to effect change. Convince a teenager that the intensive, purposeful practice is worth it and he will improve, usually by one or two levels of function. It is a golden opportunity. This period, then, is a prime opportunity to work around established maladaptive habits.

Modern Therapeutic Interventions

Managing spasticity in an older child or a teen is now possible, and several promising options are available, including botulinum toxin, selective dorsal rhizotomy, the Baclofen pump, and various orthopedic surgeries. Each of these interventions has been shown to be effective in research trials. Unfortunately, access to them is still limited. Referral to a spasticity management team depends on a referral from a neurologist or cerebral palsy expert, and sometimes that can be a bit of a challenge for the family. Most teenagers over the age of twelve have never been offered these interventions.

Orthopedic surgeries have also improved greatly at both ends of the severity spectrum. Single-Event Multilevel Surgeries have completely changed the outlook for older children and adults who did not have their spasticity and bodily distortion controlled earlier in life. At the other end of the spectrum, Selective Percutaneous Myofascial Release is usually used earlier in life, as it is a much less invasive procedure, done without requiring a surgical incision. There is no valid reason to think that this surgery could not also be offered to teens and even adults with milder but still persistent spasticity. At both ends of the age range of children with CP, there are proven, effective interventions to break up the negative spasticity feedback loop and correct biomechanical alignment. In many of the teenagers with GMFCS Levels of III or IV and even some at Level V, both spasticity management and orthopedic correction may be needed to achieve the best possible result. Again, information about and access to these interventions is often delayed or denied by my more conservative colleagues who point to the now outdated GMFCS Motor Growth Curves to justify their non-action.[6]

Gaining access to these promising treatments is a huge challenge, but parents have a good reason to work hard at it. The future holds enormous promise, as the following three stories demonstrate. One is about a sixteen-year-old young man with spastic diplegia. The second describes a rapidly growing teenager with a birth-related brachial plexus injury. The third story is about a healthy, athletic preteen who suddenly became paralyzed from the neck down. Each of these teens and their parents committed time and resources to achieve more than was expected by their healthcare teams. They prove that the future is not what it used to be.

Mason's Story

Mason has spastic diplegia, the type of cerebral palsy that primarily affects his legs. His mother, Ruth, a healthcare professional, has consistently advocated for her son. She had him doing therapy from the age of three. When he needed surgery to treat his spasticity, she got that done. Her efforts, and his, have yielded results. As a preteen he was smart and doing well at school, able to get around with a cane in each hand. But, like many, he was becoming fed up with therapy. He wanted to get on with his life.

Mason had been through several orthopedic surgeries over the years, plus a selective dorsal rhizotomy to address his spasticity. At sixteen he was generally weak, had poor alignment especially in the ankles and trunk, and consequently had poor balance. He walked with two canes. When he tried to walk without support, he was afraid of falling. He had poor body awareness, in both his trunk and legs.

He was sixteen and he was exerting his independence. He had had enough. He refused to wear his braces and he was actively refusing any suggestion of further therapy. I met him when I was giving a talk at a parent organization headed by his mother. We talked briefly after I had spoken to the group and it did not go well.

Mason didn't believe me when I said it was possible for him to improve. After all he had been through, he was not happy with the results. Therapy and all those surgeries had not made him better and now he was slowly but surely getting worse. This is a not uncommon response from teenagers and even parents who are discouraged and have lost any realistic hope for change. I asked Mason to think about it and told his mother about Pia Stampe, the physical therapist in Rochester, New York, who was happy to do short-term intensives with doubtful teenagers.

A full year later, his mother, Ruth, overriding his objections, finally persuaded him to try a one-week intensive with Pia.

It got off to a difficult start.

His mother says, "Mason is hard-headed. He had flat-out refused to wear his braces any longer. He told her that he was fine as he was." They had one week of daily three-hour sessions to work with Mason. Three therapists spent an hour each using biofeedback, supportive garments, and braces to first improve his alignment and body awareness, followed by balance training and strengthening. With every exercise, every posture, and every muscle recruitment, Mason and his mother were shown exactly what that particular thing was doing for him and how it would be better if it got stronger as he continued to work at it.

Ruth and Mason both were delighted by the changes they saw.

Mason (in his words) achieved the following in one week:

1. Improved posture
2. Head back (not chin down)
3. Balance (walking with legs instead of canes)
4. Found quad muscles
5. Decision made to wear his braces!
6. Walking with one cane (as an assist, not balance)
7. Developed a train-like-an-athlete program for home/ gym use

Ruth says, "He left *so* proud of himself and was really optimistic about what his future can hold if he works hard enough towards it. I left with regained hope and again, deep in my heart, I knew there was more."

In a one-week intensive, Mason moved from a deteriorating GMFCS Level III to almost a Level II. I have every expectation that he can move again to a Level II and even Level I if he continues to strengthen and develop new walking patterns. And if he makes it to Level I, we will change the goal and set it higher. Left without intervention, teenagers deteriorate through puberty. In contrast, if teenagers can see that change is possible, they can improve. They now have the brainpower to understand and work hard and they have a body that is actively growing.

Richard's Story

Richard was born with a brachial plexus injury. His mother, Vanda, remembers being told that he would never function well in a two-handed environment. They told her to take him home and treat him like a normal baby. Whatever recovery he achieved, they said, he would achieve on his own. Later, when he was three, the family was told that they could try some therapy. Richard is part of an athletic, motivated family, and they took an active role in all the recommended therapy exercises, strengthening, and stretches. By the time he was six years old, Richard was discharged from therapy, having achieved all the initial goals set by the therapists for his recovery. All was well until he started to grow quickly as he approached puberty. This rapid growth led to a progressive loss of function, changing the way he lifted his hand to his mouth or over his head. By the time he was ten, he had pain in his shoulder and arm. Unfortunately, there are no exceptions to the rule that unbalanced muscle pull in a growing child leads to progressive distortion and pain. Richard and his mother were motivated—Richard was hurting and frustrated by the turn his condition was taking.

I first saw Richard at age twelve. He had lost range of movement in his BPI-affected arm when he and his mother, Vanda, came to see me. He was in pain and motivated to change. Some of his loss of function was related to pubertal growth without therapy. The mild muscle imbalance he was left with when discharged from therapy at age six progressed when he started to grow rapidly. If he were a teen with CP, common wisdom would say the short, tight spastic muscles were further shortened by a failure to keep up with bone growth. But he was not spastic. The common feature in deterioration in BPI seems to be unbalanced strength and pull on the bones.

Shoulders are difficult to rehabilitate. Numerous therapy courses are available for adult shoulder problems, but to my knowledge the only shoulder-specific pediatric therapy courses were a few that I did with my friend and colleague Karen Orlando. I took Richard and Vanda to her to design a specific recovery program for him. Karen is an internationally recognized sports physiotherapist who has worked with both Olympic and Paralympic teams and for twenty years with the Canadian Rowing Team.

The first thing Karen and I noticed about Richard was the way his shoulder blades stuck out. The term for this is "winging scapula" and it's very common in children with BPI due to an imbalance between the stronger anterior rotator cuff muscles and the weaker posterior rotator cuff muscles. In Richard's case, there was massive winging of the "good" shoulder as well as the affected one. This was not caused by neurologic damage. It was the result of chronic overuse of a joint that was unable to tolerate the loads being placed upon it. His shoulders were damaged because his family did what their physiotherapist told them to do. The therapist had told them to walk him on his hands in order to strengthen his shoulders, and that's what they did. The entire family took turns helping Richard walk on his hands. This widely used exercise is called wheelbarrow walking. Wheelbarrow walking is a frequently recommended therapeutic technique in pediatric rehabilitation for strengthening the shoulder in children with BPI and cerebral palsy, although I have never found any research to back up the claims of benefit. For Richard, it was a disastrous mistake.

When we first examined him, he could only get his arm up about shoulder height, and the only way to get it above his head was with a big body swing. Karen's first reaction was that he must not have innervation to both sides or the scapula wouldn't be winging so badly. The muscles wouldn't be so weak and he would be able to lift his hand above his head. She said his triceps were terrible. He lay down on his left side on the physio table and stuck his elbow straight up in the air with his hand hanging down towards his shoulder. Orlando asked him to use his triceps to extend his hand to the ceiling and he couldn't do it. Not at all. He couldn't even lift the weight of his own hand up.

We started him with TES in the hope of getting some muscle growth and got him a shoulder brace to hold his arm in the shoulder joint. Full dislocation, or more commonly posterior subluxation of the shoulder, is very common in children with BPI. One early shoulder MRI study demonstrated this problem as early as six months of age.[7] If there is muscle weakness, then the place to start is by treating the weakness in proper alignment. Functional change, which so often is the first issue addressed in therapy, should come after alignment.

Function follows form in both unaffected athletes and teens with neurologic damage.

Vanda recalls, "He had to wear a shoulder brace every day. We had him splinted at night and strapped up to keep him in the proper position. It was a progressive splinting system because his elbow had started to contract to where he couldn't even straighten it all the way. The triceps was so weak that the biceps was overpowering it and it was causing a contracture so he couldn't straighten his arm anymore. He also couldn't supinate, where you put your hands in front of you and you have your palms to the floor and then turn your palms to the ceiling."

Richard and his parents had to make a significant commitment in order to implement the regime I set up for them. Richard put up with considerable discomfort and expended a lot of effort. His parents put time and financial resources into making things happen. It took a couple of years to bring about significant change.

"It was astounding. He extended his arm with a five-pound weight on it," says Vanda. "He could get his palm to the ceiling and he could get his hand to his mouth without his elbow going out to the side. He could lift his hand completely above his head against resistance. He couldn't even lift it up before. The shoulder blades tightened up and came into his body and his posture improved. He had less pain and just so many things that everyone said that there was no way he could do those movements, let alone do them with resistance. It was the strength training. Yes, it was astounding.

"Most people do not know that there is anything wrong with him. When he stands, his elbow is a little bit crooked but it is not noticeable to people unless you are a physiotherapist. Most people don't know that he has any disability at all. He went on to make his grade ten volleyball team. He could get his hands above his head to block and serve."

Richard and his mother showed what could be achieved through intensive therapy if only the right thing is done at the right time in the right order.

If Mason needed to be convinced that intensive work, starting with conditioning and alignment, was in his best interest, Richard and his mother had no doubts.

Vanda sums it up. "Dr. Pape was all about brain plasticity and working with the person like you would an athlete. You can take a couch potato and if you start actually working the muscles you can turn them into an athlete. She just takes those same principles and applies them to people starting with disabilities and recovers the muscles. Richard won't ever be a world-class weight lifter, but his improvement from where he was at to well within normal functioning range is the equivalent of taking a normally functioning person and turning them into super strong."

Julie's Story

Julie was eleven years old when she was struck down. She first felt a pain in her left arm. It spread across her back and then kept spreading until, within in an hour, she collapsed and was taken to the hospital. She was admitted to the ICU and ventilated, as by then, she was completely paralyzed and unable to breathe on her own. An MRI showed that her upper spine was inflamed, leading to a diagnosis of transverse myelitis, triggered by a rare virus.

Once they had the diagnosis, Julie was given a series of three plasma exchanges over a period of six days. Nothing much happened after the first one, but a few hours after the second one, a young doctor thought he saw her toe twitch. She was four weeks in the ICU, and then two weeks in the neurology ward. By the time they discharged her, she was breathing independently, eating soft food, and had some movement in her lower limbs. The doctors sent her to Bloorview Holland Rehabilitation Hospital with encouraging words for her continued recovery. They kept to themselves what they really thought, which was that Julie would never walk again.

Bloorview takes in a wide variety of children with a range of disabilities. The staff do their best to meet their patients' needs, but those needs vary enormously: some are in for a short period to give their family respite; others are long-term residents with nowhere else to go. Julie had two hours of therapy per day, five days a week. Slowly she recovered. She went from wheelchair to walker.

The doctor who saw her move her toe for the first time back at Sick Kids saw her at Bloorview before she was discharged, walking in a walker. He said, "Remember me from ICU? I saw you move your toe. Now look at you! I can't believe it. This is great." Julie did not think that was enough, but even though he saw her progress, he said, "I don't know if you will be able to go beyond a walker." Julie said, "I am going to do what I can."

When Bob and Sue introduced me to their daughter, Julie had some doubts about my initial recommendation. Throughout her illness she had been cautioned to not expect too much. This was well-intentioned advice, but it discouraged hope in both Julie and her family.

Sue remembers, "Karen met Julie and said, 'I will work with you but I want you to do as I say. I will be your coach, and remember no pressure, no diamonds.' Julie, age twelve, said, 'Yes, pressure! Yes, diamonds! I want to get better.'"

When I examined Julie, I wanted first to deal with her general weakness, especially as it affected her trunk, and consequently her breathing. I saw that her respiratory function was poor. She had not been given any breathing exercises to do after her weeks on a ventilator and I felt this was the best place to start her program. I asked her to start jogging in a Wet Vest and to do yoga. I could tell she thought I was crazy, but I asked her to do these exercises for a month and then come back.

Her mother found a physiotherapist/personal trainer who specialized in yoga training. She did yoga a couple of times a week and had a list of home exercises that she would do every day. Julie did yoga deep-breathing exercises and after a month, she increased her respiratory capacity by two inches when comparing a full inspiration to full exhalation.

Julie and her family came back and said, "Dr. Pape, we are on board."

After several years and multiple interventions, Julie is running again, swimming, and has regained significant use of her fingers. Her illness is a rare one and we do not have any real idea if she will regain all that she lost. But I do know that there are no data to support the *no hope* prognosis that her family was given. I am proud of her and her parents for not believing her doctors when they told her she would be wheelchair-bound for life.

— • —

The relationship between the doctor or therapist and the patient, like the relationship between an athlete and coach, is important. If the patient has no faith that the therapist's instructions will bring about positive change, she's unlikely to comply with them. She just won't do the work. How often do we see top-level athletes fire a coach when they find themselves on a losing streak? It's exactly the same if a young person with cerebral palsy decides that he's on a losing streak. The therapist is ignored or fired.

Therapists also have their preferences. Some are happier working with younger children than with older ones. Cindy Servello, an experienced occupational therapist with a special interest in infants with brachial plexus injury, works effectively with both age groups but she acknowledges the difficulty. "I do treat older children but I don't like it. It is the truth because it's harder. Karen has always said, and I have this in my head, it takes thousands of repetitions to make any change. Who has time for thousands of perfect repetitions? You do therapy, and you get a good result in therapy, and then you look out the window and they're doing it wrong again. Changing a habit is very difficult."

Christine Egan, another experienced physical therapist, takes a different view: "I actually like working with older kids because at some point they become personally invested in what they are doing.... I think they want to be better personally. It is not somebody else wanting them to be better. It is more of an internal motivation. Not doing it for Daddy, or whatever."

There has never been a time like the present in the world of pediatric neurorehabilitation. Many of the current leaders in pediatric rehabilitation agree. Iona Novak sums up the possibilities, saying, "There are now at least sixty-four different interventions for cerebral palsy[8] with even more interventions being studied at clinical trial." It's time to raise our expectations by setting higher goals for rehabilitation.

"For years there has been much appropriate sensitivity about not trying to make children with CP 'normal,' because that has not yet been thought possible," physiotherapist Diane Damiano writes. "But what if it were possible to make a child with Cerebral Palsy walk like any other child? The evidence gives us every reason to be optimistic about this grand goal."[9]

As Mason, Richard, and Julie show, change is possible. My own experience, caring for thousands of children with CP, shows that children can improve or even function within what we consider to be normal limits. I have seen children at GMFCS Levels I and II function well within the normal range, and there is hope for significant improvement in all but the small proportion of the most severely affected children in Level V.

For most teens with CP, it is not too late to get better. They have a great opportunity to grow and heal while their brains and bodies are growing at an extraordinary pace. They need a new type of therapy based on an athletic model. Doing more of the same old, same old harder will definitely not work. They need to be treated like a world-class athlete. They need measurable, achievable short-term goals and a rigorous training schedule that is both challenging and, more importantly, fun.

Our educational system should start to provide these teenagers with modified class schedules that allow time for daily training. This accommodation is provided for skilled musicians, actors, and junior athletes to work on their skills. Children with a brain or nerve injury deserve the same consideration. Finishing high school may take a bit longer than the usual four years, but what a difference it would make for the rest of their life if they are able to walk unaided into their college or university career. Another option is for them to do a gap year after high school to do intensive training. It also works, but it is harder. For many, the chief problem they will face is access to the therapies that are shown to work or are at least promising. If they can access modern interventions, you will see, they can get a whole lot better.

fourteen

It Is Never Too Late to Change

What hope is there for an adult who has lived with cerebral palsy all his life? Most pediatric hospitals and clinics have firm guidelines that oblige them to discharge patients when they're eighteen or, at the latest, twenty-one. Most patients leave formal therapy long before they graduate from high school. There are only a few physicians or surgeons who provide care for older individuals with cerebral palsy or brachial plexus injury. Most of the care that is provided comes from a small number of pediatric cerebral palsy specialists who also see adult patients. This is good as far as it goes, but these specialists are first and foremost pediatricians or pediatric orthopedic surgeons. In most areas, there is no organized way for adult patients to access and benefit from all the new techniques and therapies that are now available to children. It is equally difficult for them to access the new treatments that have been developed in the adult world for people with stroke or spinal cord injury. As we have noted repeatedly, the adult medical community is much further advanced in its understanding of neuroplasticity as it applies to stroke patients and other later-onset neurologic problems. Great progress is being made in other areas but not for survivors of early neurologic injury.

This is a growing social and medical problem. Of the roughly one million people in the United States with cerebral palsy, more than half are adults without adequate healthcare. The specialists they need to deliver twenty-first-century neurorehabilitation are just not available. This population of adults can be accurately described as therapeutic orphans. It is a growing problem as happily, the death rate of children with early brain damage is now close to that of the general population.[1] Each year, more eighteen- to twenty-year-olds are kicked out of the pediatric healthcare system.

Adults with cerebral palsy face other obstacles. They have had a lifetime to firmly wire in their abnormal habits. Because they have never experienced normal movement, most find it hard to even imagine moving differently. Their habits are deeply embedded, and consequently they're that much harder to work around. Plus adults can no longer benefit from the peak periods of neuroplasticity seen in small children and teenagers.

But adulthood has its advantages too. Neuroplasticity lasts a lifetime: the brain never stops changing, growing, and adapting to challenge. The same treatments and therapies that work for younger patients can work for adults. And adults do have an edge over their younger counterparts in this respect: all (or most) of the complicated issues revolving around independence and growth have been resolved. Adults are likely to be strongly motivated and they have the ability, once focused, to concentrate on a task.

Norah's Story

Norah has mild spastic diplegia, cerebral palsy affecting both her legs. Her mother, Barbara, first brought her to me at the Magee Clinic when she was six years old. She did TES, stretching, and a variety of other therapies to strengthen her legs and improve her gait. She had surgery to correct the alignment of one leg when she was eleven and was discharged from therapy, as many children are, when she reached a plateau at thirteen. She was walking independently. She was able to take up dance "for the love of it," she says, "rather than technical ability" when she was in her teens. She worked out regularly at the gym and swam. She was smart, active, conscientious, and always willing to work hard. In the summer of 2007, she went to England to study and walked everywhere. She didn't think she was exercising or doing therapy, but she got better. When her parents and sister came to visit, they immediately noticed that her body was different—it was straighter.

Norah returned from England to continue her undergraduate program at the University of Winnipeg. When she and her mother came to see me in Toronto, we talked about developing a program for her that would build on the improvement she had achieved on her own. Over the course of the next year or so, Norah came to see me periodically to review and upgrade her program.

She describes the program as follows. "So we met Dr. Pape and she said that I could get better and this was the first time we had heard that my disability could be overcome. It could actually get better; it was something that I could improve on. She gave us a choice of a bunch of things like martial arts, yoga, physio, Pilates, and training in the gym. Then I met with Karen Orlando, and had a massage with a therapist that Karen referred me to.

"It was very difficult for me because I didn't fully believe it, I didn't feel it in my body, and you can only stay motivated with something if you believe that it's possible. At the beginning, I just did gym-based training and I went to the pool. I wore a Wet Vest in the pool and the difference was ... I hate the word 'normal,' but in this context it normalizes your gait pattern. If you jog in the water with the Wet Vest and if you do it enough in the water, your body starts to adapt to it when you're on land. With the Wet Vest I felt more supported. I was jogging and doing stuff with barbells in the water. And then I started doing yoga, trying out some yoga poses in the water, and I found that I could actually hold balancing yoga poses in the water that I couldn't when I was in the yoga studio. If I did them in the pool, I could hold them, but if I did them in the studio I would fall over.

"Karen Orlando helped me with my walk, woke up my feet and had me doing stretches for my hip flexors. I still don't feel it in my gait. I feel it in my body. I think that I started to believe when I started Pilates. I really enjoy Pilates and I felt like I wasn't fighting through the therapy and I wasn't fighting with my body. I felt like I was working with my body. So I was a lot more motivated to do it. Pilates is about core strength and balance and this is the thing, the feedback I got from people with that, my pelvis was less twisted. I was more open in my chest. My spine was a lot straighter, my legs were a lot straighter, and my overall balance was a lot better."

After Norah completed her undergraduate degree, she moved to Toronto and took courses at Ryerson. I told her that if she wanted to move up a level, to really change her condition, she needed to devote more time to it. I suggested that she consider taking time off from her studies and undertake an intensive. We used the term "boot camp" as a way of representing the kind of intensity she needed to bring to training. We enlisted Karen Orlando to direct Norah's program.

"I decided to study publishing in Toronto and to take a couple of courses at Ryerson and the rest of the time I devoted to working at Karen Orlando's clinic," Norah recalls. "So I went to Karen Orlando's every day and did physio and massage and Pilates. I did at least two hours a day, five days a week.

"My body and walk have changed to the point that people who have known me for years don't recognize me. There are times when my mother doesn't recognize me walking towards her. My next-door neighbour told me last summer that there are times when he doesn't recognize me walking past his house or down the street. He said I not only walk differently, but I carry myself completely differently. He told me, 'Whatever you're doing, it's working.'"

Erik's Story

Spastic diplegia was a central part of Erik's childhood. His parents were great advocates and insisted that he have surgeries, therapy, and treatments like patterning. But after high school he left most of that behind him to concentrate on launching his career. He got married and had children. He worked out regularly and had a demanding job. By the time he was forty-eight, it had been years since he had given much thought or attention to the disabilities that had disrupted his youth.

But then things started happening.

"My knee was occasionally very painful for weeks at a time and would sometimes give out on me," says Erik. "My hip would spasm or my back would seize up. Being in crowds or around small children or animals made me nervous, as quick movements in my vicinity would upset my balance and sometimes make me fall. I fell in public more often than I wanted, and I hated the stares and even the kind questions from people wanting to help. I had the discouraging feeling that a lot of people never saw past my disability.

"But when I sought help for injuries, doctors seemed to look only at the body part that was bothering me and never at how my body worked as a whole. I occasionally saw a physical therapist and got massages, and Pilates helped a lot. Twice I called the cerebral palsy clinic at the children's hospital where I live, but I was told they don't see adult patients. I knew I needed something more, but I had no idea where to find it.

"The professionals I saw talked about managing my symptoms, but no one ever suggested that I could vastly improve the way my body worked and alleviate many of the symptoms of CP. I was left with the impression that things would slowly get worse, despite my efforts to stay in good shape. Last year my back spasms were so bad that I would collapse and spend days in bed. A doctor I saw said that decades of tight muscles and a choppy gait had taken a toll on my body and I could expect problems like this to start occurring more often.

"I couldn't accept that prognosis. I was forty-eight. My wife and I had plans to travel after our kids were grown. I want an active, healthy retirement. I plan to exercise and work for many years to come."

Then Erik's wife discovered my website. "It was the first time either of us had ever heard the idea that the movements associated with CP were habits and that new habits could be learned, even for a middle-aged adult," says Erik.

I sent him to see Pia Stampe in Rochester, New York. He completed a three-day intensive course at Pia's clinic, Step by Step Therapy Center. "Erik's assessment revealed that he had significant tightness in spastic muscle groups combined with overall weakness in his legs and hips," Pia says. "The tightness and weakness impacted Erik's gait, balance, and coordination. The intervention focused on creating a home program that would help Erik regain range of motion, strengthen weak muscles, and improve overall balance and coordination. Erik's home program included a water training program and he was started on TES to address his weak and atrophied [wasted] muscles."

"Pia was the first person that seemed to look at my body as a whole and could explain how, for instance, tightness in my pelvis cascaded into difficulty with my gait and pain in different parts of my body," says Erik.

After a thorough assessment, Erik got down to work with Pia. "I wish everyone could experience the feeling I had on the mat when, within a relatively short period, my legs and pelvis were put in a more relaxed position than they have ever been," says Erik. "It was a euphoric relief, and it felt like a hardened crust being removed from my body. Each long breath in a darkened, quiet room, with Pia's firm and gentle hands rocking my muscles as if I were an infant, brought on a wave of relief. While I knew I had very spastic muscles, I never knew that a slow and systematic rocking of the muscles could prepare me minutes later to stand straighter than I ever have.

"The release was more than just in my tight muscles, though. The release was letting go of the years of frustration and coping. The moments as a child when I worked so hard to be included in many activities. It was the release of feelings about the frozen stares from strangers trying to figure out what must be wrong with me. The embarrassment of falling in public places and not wanting the attention from those who offer help. The memories of frustrating trips to doctors as a kid when I was told to come back later when they could do surgery. It was all there leaking out from my body and into the mat.

"Then came the tears."

In my experience, most people with a disability reach a point where they have had enough of therapy. They accommodate to their level of impairment and get on with life. Norah went to Europe the first time with the primary idea of being a tourist and seeing as much as she could in a limited time. She walked miles and improved. Erik was active and athletic, but he had no specific routine adapted to his condition. He needed, but wasn't getting, the massage and stretching that are considered routine and indispensable for most serious athletes: it's how the body rests and recovers from exertion. Walking for many with CP is hard work and they too need rest and regeneration routines.

"We worked on gait training," Erik says, "and created a long-term plan to build on our initial accomplishments, a plan that includes heat, massage, stretching, gym, and water exercises. We have a long-term goal of using Botox and taking advantage of lessened spasticity to strengthen my muscles.

"Now, my fitness and my activities are done with greater purpose. Each day brings a little reminder of how things are different, like how my feet now sound different hitting the floor. Friends and colleagues say already that I look taller, and I have a looseness that I've never had before. My body and mind are ready for the work, and I am eager to see how much progress I can make.

"I still go to the gym most mornings and ride the bike and lift weights. I still eat well and drink lots of water. There are, however, lots of things that are different. There are moments where certain parts of my new regimen seem to be having the most impact and times when other practices seem more significant. Some parts of the routine are rewarding and others are inconvenient. My thought is that it does not matter what is having the greatest impact; what matters is that I believe in the entire protocol.

"I sit through assisted stretches that allow me to stand straighter than I can ever remember. I sit daily in the Nada chair [a chair designed to give therapeutic back support] for thirty minutes. I go to the warm-water pool regularly, and have a specific program I follow when I get there. There is an increased awareness of how my body works.

"I'm thrilled to report that I have not fallen down since the intensive almost three months ago. I used to fall down every other week."

Christine's Story

Christine is an accomplished young woman with choreoathetosis, a severe type of cerebral palsy involving all four limbs. She was diagnosed at an early age and had years of therapy that succeeded in helping her to achieve independence and an active career. Her movements, however, remained largely uncontrolled and she spoke with difficulty. After she graduated from university, she started a not-for-profit organization, Kids Are Kids, visiting primary school classrooms to talk about the experience of growing up with cerebral palsy. She found that at first the children were uncomfortable with her. Most had never met an adult with a speech impairment and difficulty controlling her movements. But Christine is a born actor and she rapidly got the children interacting with her. Her goal was to demystify disabilities. She travelled to schools throughout the Philadelphia area to provide this program. Later, after attending a summer drama camp, she started Acting Without Boundaries, a drama program for children and adults with disabilities.

Christine was physically competent and could swim after a fashion. She could do some complicated yoga poses and had been attending Pilates mat classes. She also tried for many years to hit a tennis ball, a family practice. She could hit it if the ball was fed to her slowly, in the right place. In each of these tasks, her skill level was higher than her walking, which was abnormal and unbalanced. When she was thirty-four she had a bad fall in which she damaged her SI (sacroiliac) joint, leaving her with persistent pain when she walked. I had known her and her family for years—our families both vacationed in Florida and we saw one another each winter. When I suggested to Christine that she could achieve real improvement if she started an intensive followed by a continuing regime of focused exercise, she initially expressed interest. Her mother and older brother were keen.

Christine had one big advantage over many adults in a comparable situation. Thanks to the diligent work of her mother and multiple therapists over the years, her body was in good alignment. People with dyskinesia, of which choreoathetosis is one form, tend to have balanced increased tone; alignment is not as much of a problem as proprioception and overall body awareness.

When it came time to start on the intensive, Christine had second thoughts. She said when she went into primary schools and the children had difficulty understanding her, her hard-to-follow speech pattern was part of who she was as a person. She's a natural actor and this was something she used to engage their attention: she would get them laughing and having fun. She said, "Who would I be if I could speak well?"

This idea, that her random movements and hard-to-follow way of speaking were part of her identity, was one factor that gave her pause. She also had years of rehabilitation behind her and had been disappointed many times. Fear of the unknown and reluctance to face another disappointing outcome are common features in the adult born with an early neurologic problem. It took courage, a leap of faith, and strong support from her family for Christine finally to accept what I had proposed.

We launched our intensive early one morning in the pool. I had decided to start by having her jog in deep water while wearing a Wet Vest. Her abnormal gait—she habitually led with her left foot and dragged her right foot behind it—was a deeply wired-in habit. But once she was in the water, her movements became normal. This was a novel, challenging task with consequences: she had to learn to stay straight in the water while moving forward. All four limbs had to work in a reciprocal manner or she would find herself going in circles. She worked as hard at the task as I asked her to, and over a three-month period, working out six days a week, she made remarkable progress. We moved her to the shallow end, so her feet touched bottom, and attached small flotation weights to her legs to increase the workload and improve her body awareness. When she was steady enough, we got her to practise "perfect walking" with a buoyant walking pole for guidance. She practised turning her trunk, another new challenge, as she walked.

This is her description: "I practise perfect walking in the pool. Experiencing perfect walking is an amazing feeling. To me, the water is freedom. I can learn to do things in the water and then I learn to do them on land. The water program has improved my walking, talking, and eating. Eating always was very difficult for me, but after doing exercises with the barbell in the water, I see a huge difference in my ability to control my arms. I can see such a difference after I swim. I love starting my day with swimming because it helps me start the day in a positive way. Water definitely is healing for everyone."

Christine hints at a key difference in the rehabilitation of an adult after a stroke and an adult who has lived with the results of a brain injury for decades. An older person with CP has never experienced what it feels like to move as the rest of us do. Water allows her to experience freer movement, and for the first time she understands what all the therapists were trying to achieve. She now knows what it feels like to do perfect walking. Equally, Erik did not know what relaxed muscles felt like until he had experienced relaxed muscles.

When I was satisfied that she was ready, I shifted practice to dry land. Initially, she used a walker. In most cases, additional support is needed while learning a new habit. Christine had been walking independently with her old habit, but now we wanted her to practise a normal pattern, replicating what she had been doing in the pool.

She was, not surprisingly, unsteady. Her gait was normal, though it didn't feel normal to her. She continued to use the walker over the course of the nine months following the first winter intensive and gradually got steadier. She was ready now—and eager—for a second intensive when we met in Florida again.

It was time to transition her to less support. I introduced her to Nordic walking poles and suggested that she practise on the beach. Christine had never been able to walk on sand. I thought this would be a powerful goal to motivate her. Walking in sand is a challenge, and our brains, which get lazy performing familiar tasks, respond well to anything new and unexpected. Her weight-training coach accompanied her on her first time out. The sand would provide a soft surface for landing on if she fell down, but we wanted her to have the confidence of knowing that help was at hand. When she tried to walk with a single pole, without her coach holding her hand, she promptly reverted to the old habit, leading with her left foot and swinging the right one up to join it.

Apparently one pole was not enough and so she tried two. Now whenever she lost the new movement pattern, she learned to stop, refocus, do a few mini-squats to help activate the correct muscle groups, and start over again.

In addition to reconstructing her walking pattern, I gave Christine other work to do, for awareness, strengthening, and ultimately improved function. She had been doing Pilates mat workouts and I got her to use the reformer instead. On the mat, there was too much freedom of motion. Using the reformer, the pulleys and springs helped keep her in perfect posture while she worked on building muscle strength. Continued water exercise improved her breath control and trunk strength. And then, to keep her motivated and making measureable progress, we put it all together on the tennis court. All programs need an element of fun.

I asked Debby, her pro, to work on her forehand volley. Debby didn't want to and her reluctance was not entirely unwarranted: Christine took a few balls in the face. The consequence of moving slowly! But this is what learning consists of: babies fall repeatedly as they practise gross motor skills, learning to stand and then walk. An older child, learning to ride a bicycle, is likely to pick up some bruises along the way. Too often children with disabilities are protected when they should be allowed to fail in the course of learning a new skill. Our brains work best when there is a problem to solve.

Once she became expert at the net, hitting up to twenty forehand volleys in a row, we moved her back from the net and started one-step mini-squat drills at mid-court. Within weeks she had moved to a one-two-three mini-squat, hit-the-ball routine. It was a novel drill. It was definitely a challenge, and the consequences included not only missing the ball but also falling down. Christine took her lumps and progressed at an amazing pace.

She returned home to Philadelphia in the spring and reported that it was a bit more of a struggle to maintain her workouts at the same level, but she did her best and held her gains. By the end of her intensives, she could eat a plate of pasta and drink a glass of wine flawlessly. She was able to work with renewed energy and was interviewed on national television about Acting Without Boundaries on the *Today Show*. Proving, after all, that her CP-related behaviour was not an essential part of her identity. She was still the person she had always been.

A Few Final Thoughts about Pain

Most teens and adults eventually run into problems with chronic pain, either as a result of progressive musculoskeletal distortion or a new injury, as Christine had. They had a chronic neurologic problem but were unable to get the attention and pain management that we all expect when we're injured or as we age. Part of the problem is that the discomfort, in most cases, grows slowly over time. It's seen as part-and-parcel of their condition. Another friend and colleague gave me insight into how this happens—how children with a chronic condition experience pain.

Richard Gross is a pediatric orthopedic surgeon in Charleston, South Carolina, with a long-time interest in children with a congenital clubfoot. The early management to correct the deformity is well established and includes casting, surgery, and therapy. Dick and I had talked about what I was doing with TES and we designed a protocol to test it in some of the children he treated. Because clubfoot is associated with abnormalities in the muscles of the lower leg, Dick wondered if TES might improve the muscle function once serial casting and/or surgery had created some ankle mobility. The study was positive overall and pointed to the conclusion that "low intensity electrical stimulation is of value for selected patients with resistant clubfoot following surgery, especially when not accompanied by fixed bony deformity."[2]

Dick's thorough patient-assessment and record-keeping routines made him an ideal research partner. Whenever he examined a patient at his clinic, he took the time to gather a detailed history and take photographs. This meant we had access to the natural history of each child's motor function over several years prior to the study.

One day, a boy included in the TES study told him that his foot didn't hurt anymore. Dick was puzzled and a little shocked because he didn't recall the boy ever having told him that his foot hurt, an observation that was confirmed when he checked his records. The boy had repeatedly, over years, said that his clubfoot did not hurt. He asked the boy why he hadn't told him about the pain before. The child answered cheerily, "I didn't know it hurt until it stopped."

When Dick told me the story, I realized that it had not occurred to me that if a child has always hurt, he may think of it simply as normal sensation, the way his body always feels. From that time forward, I changed the way I talked to children and teenagers about pain. I would ask them if there was anything different about the way their two shoulders felt. I would ask whether there was a difference between their hands or if their leg felt different over the course of the day. Richard, the teenager with BPI, initially told me that he felt no pain in his affected shoulder and arm. I asked him if he ever had to take an Advil or Tylenol to ease an ache. Sure, he said, but only when it was really bad. I showed him a pain scale, a chart that assigns a number corresponding to the intensity of pain, in which 1 is scarcely noticeable and 10 is unbearable. When he looked at the chart, he started to understand what I was getting at. I asked him to compare his two sides. He said the unaffected side didn't hurt unless he had an injury. His affected shoulder and arm were a level 2 to 4 all the time! He only asked for a pain pill when the BPI side felt like a 7 to 10. On an everyday basis, he said, the BPI side was always different from the other side. It varied from a 2 on the best days to a 5 or 6 by the end of a hard or active day. It turns out that when asking a child about pain, we have to ask the right questions to get the right answer.

— • —

Cerebral palsy is thought of chiefly as a condition that affects children and almost all the resources that are available are directed at children. But cerebral palsy, like brachial plexus injury and spinal cord damage, is for life. The initial injury may be a one-time event, but the secondary effects are progressive and the adults require attention.

Norah, Erik, and Christine all found therapy that changed their lives in a positive way. It wasn't easy. Erik was actually turned away from institutions dedicated to treating his condition—but not his age group. Norah and her mother had to travel halfway across the continent to find the help they wanted. It was purely by chance that I found Christine. The techniques that brought change in each of these individuals were similar and, by now, familiar to readers. What works for children and adolescents also worked for them. The challenge now is to make these therapies available to all who need them.

Over the years, I have treated adults with varying degrees of physical impairment. Their willingness to work and their determination, combined with adherence to a daily program that incorporated these principles, made a significant change in the way they live their lives. It—really—is never too late.

fifteen

Aim for a Cure

After a brain injury at or near birth, we now know that children's brains recover. Their brains heal and grow, and they gain the ability to do far more than we expect. The boy can run even if he can't walk properly. The girl who cannot lift her arms can do jumping jacks. The teenager who walks awkwardly can tap dance beautifully. They can do this because their brains have recovered—the same part of the brain that directs the action of walking. Yet, as we have seen, the awkward walking patterns persist because they're bad habits, a holdover from the time when their brains were still healing.

Most doctors and therapists don't see this potential in children with CP. It took me a long time to understand why. Part of the problem was the very human failing of seeing what we expect to see and ignoring, or dismissing, what we do not expect to see. What the doctor or therapist sees is one of the characteristic patterns of cerebral palsy and the body distortion that results from adapting to spasticity, or the arm and hand positions found in children that are so typical of a persistent brachial plexus injury. These are maladaptive movement habits combined with muscle weakness, and they hide the real story—the extent of the child's brain recovery.

The real potential of these children is easy to miss, even for the expert. If you're a doctor or therapist, and you see a child walking with an awkward gait, it's understandable that you might not ask him to run down the hall. Yet it happens all the time. At a cerebral palsy meeting a few years ago, an experienced pediatric orthopedic surgeon came up to me and said, "All my kids with hemiplegia run better than they walk, I just never understood what it meant." There are countless examples to demonstrate that the skills acquired early when the brain was damaged can conceal later recovery if we restrict our focus to seeing what we expect to see—such as the abnormal walk that defines the diagnosis of cerebral palsy.

I had the same problem for many years. Even though I had been taught about human neuroplasticity early in my career and I saw examples of full recovery in babies with documented brain damage, it took years of experience in different silos of pediatric care before I started to see what was right in front of me. Until I examined a wide range of children of all ages with a wide variety of brain, spinal cord, and nerve injuries, I too thought that spasticity in early brain injuries was only related to the child's brain damage. This may be true in adult forms of spasticity, but in children, a very significant part of what is called spasticity is actually a side effect.

As I have argued in this book, much of spasticity is a habit of the brain and body. It begins when the brain is damaged and the baby tries to move against gravity. The nerves send a signal to the muscles that are easiest to activate—the flexor muscles of the upper body and the extensor muscles of the lower body. These muscles inhibit the muscles that are supposed to be their partners in creating a fluid movement, and in doing so they destroy the elegant dance that most of us take for granted. Every time the child tries to move a hand or stand up, the bully muscles get stronger and the partner muscles get weaker. Eventually, after thousands of repetitions, it forms a facilitated network in the brain that guides the awkward movement. I call this a negative feedback loop, and it springs into action every time the person wants to move. Eventually it may distort bones and joints, which causes further problems. This theory explains why spasticity gets worse in children with CP, even though their brain damage occurred at or near birth and didn't happen again.

There are two important conclusions. The first is that side effects can be prevented in some and treated in others. We need to be far more proactive in the pediatric neurorehabilitation world. We should be diagnosing the babies who are *at risk* far earlier.[1] Unfortunately, when I make this sort of comment, the hackles of the steadfast defenders of the past rear up. A recent letter to the editor of the journal *Pediatrics* encapsulates this traditionalist position. After discussing the perils of early prediction of later neurologic handicap based on brain scans in the neonatal period, a respected, senior neonatologist writes, "We need to understand the potential impact of our predictive uncertainty on the parents of these vulnerable infants [*with an abnormality diagnosed on an early brain scan*]."[2] In the research study that sparked his comments, a significant proportion, roughly a quarter of the study population with severe abnormalities on their brain scan, were only mildly impaired or unimpaired at follow-up examinations at eighteen to twenty-two months of age.

This is the same old story. The experts worry about making a "mistake." They continue to deny that the brain scans were abnormal, but the baby recovered. This is a cause for celebration, not silly arguments about "protecting" parents from the potential of bad news. They seem to honestly believe that parents would rather be told their child has an abnormality evident on the brain scan, but they do not have anything to do about it until some time in the future. If the baby grows up with abnormal movements, then we will start treatment when they are *bad enough.*

It really is time to change. I can think of no other area of pediatric healthcare where early treatment is not given with the hope of preventing or lessening any deterioration. Yes, Mrs. Jones, little Katie does have a bad cough and her chest X-ray shows an abnormality that *might* develop into a serious pneumonia, but I think we should *wait and see* what happens before we talk about starting treatment.

The second important conclusion is that side effects are treatable. You do not have to believe in neuroplasticity. You just need to access and use the evidence-informed and best-practice treatments that are available at the right time, and in the right order. In most situations, earlier treatment is better than later.

Why isn't this happening? It's not for a lack of good will. Everyone who works with children with cerebral palsy wants to make their lives better. A generation ago, when most children with CP had its most severe forms, the prospects for recovery were not good. Those severely affected children were likely to have a degree of permanent physical and cognitive dysfunction. A generation ago, we didn't know about the brain's remarkable ability to change, so we were operating on the premise that brain damage was permanent and irreversible. It made sense for healthcare providers working with children with CP to take the view that we had to be realistic: therapists, then, did not seek to instil normal behaviour patterns in their patients; they just tried to keep the children as comfortable as possible and stop them from getting worse. Families, and everyone trying to help children with cerebral palsy, were supposed to accept physical limitations, abandon the idea of what's normal or abnormal, and cherish CP children in spite of the disabilities that make their lives difficult.

This was, at the time, a humane approach to the treatment of children with early brain damage.

But times have changed. Human neuroplasticity is no longer a theory. The brain's remarkable ability to change and heal is now the foundation of modern care for adults who have suffered strokes. We know baby brains can recover too. Just look at all the documented cases of babies who had serious brain injury at birth and just a couple of years later were running and playing like any other child, with no evidence of cognitive problems. Their brains recovered.

Today, over 80 percent of diagnosed children have a mild version of cerebral palsy—Level I, II, or III on the GMFCS assessment. With new techniques inspired by the neuroplasticity revolution, most of them can reasonably expect to improve by at least one level. In my experience, a good number can learn to walk and move in a way that looks like anyone without brain damage. As for the children with more severe problems, one-quarter of the total, most can also improve their functional abilities with up-to-date approaches. Even adults can improve their function, despite a lifetime of maladaptive physical habits.

This is a real, not false, hope. Surely, given the opportunities we have now, we should do what is possible to replace maladaptive function with behaviour that gives the child the opportunity to be as mobile and pain-free as his peers. We now have the tools, the skills, and insight to do this. We have come to a place where the old paradigm is no longer viable. The evidence that the brain can change and heal is in. The human examples are there for all to see, and there are so many of them that they can no longer be dismissed as outliers. There are too many boys who can run but not walk.

Children, and even adults with CP, should be given the chance to improve their physical functions and avoid the lifetime of pain that so often accompanies the physical impairments. Changing bad habits is hard work, it's true, and some parents, older children, and adults will not be willing to put in the work to change. That's fine. But making a choice without clearly understanding both the available options and the predictable consequences of their choices is wrong. To not even offer the therapies that are proven to work is a denial of care.

It's time for a change, and change doesn't come easily.

I've described what it took to bring me to my present understanding of a baby's neurologic resilience: the observations, investigations, and anomalies that, over a period of decades, led me away from the outworn theory that the parts of the infant brain that control motor function, once injured, inevitably lead to a permanent disorder of function, and that there's nothing to be done. It took a spirited five-year-old struggling to sit for the first time; a seven-year-old boy who inexplicably played soccer; a little girl of the same age who, suddenly and unexpectedly, clapped her hands above her head; and so many others, a virtual parade of infants, toddlers, preteens, and youths, demonstrating that children, young and old, even adults, all have neuroplasticity. It took all that and more, including the advice of colleagues, research from other disciplines, any number of ingenious therapists, and my tennis coach, to push me to a new way of thinking about early brain and nerve injury.

Doctors and therapists need to recognize what I have seen, that it's possible to help children with CP to improve because much of their problems are actually bad habits. But even that won't solve the problem. One of the problems, as we have seen, is that most of the CP experts see only one part of the story. The system is defined by the age of the child, so no one, apart from the pediatrician, sees the child with CP grow up. The result is that most of the experts in the system do not have the chance to see the whole picture, with both the challenges and opportunities for growth and improvement that occur throughout a child's life.

Parents, however, do. I now believe that the best results in children with CP happen when they have pushy parents who demand active intervention. In a medical world where doctors stick to their specific specialties, parents are the only constant presence in their child's life. They are the best hope for change.

So what should parents be demanding of their health-care providers? The evidence is in that habits do not change with traditional therapy, but coaches, athletes, and neuroscientists know habits can be replaced using novel, challenging tasks. If we all work together to discover more ways for children to practise new skills while having fun, the improvements will be greater and come at a faster rate.

The big problem, of course, is spasticity. As we've seen, much of it is treatable because it is not, as doctors once thought, directly linked to irreversible brain damage.

What are the treatments and therapies that make sense when these theories are understood? We've barely begun to explore the possibilities.

Prevention comes first. A habit can be prevented or lessened by addressing weakness and alignment before dysfunctional movement patterns are established. Stretching, massage, supportive garments, wrist/hand splints, and AFOs are a place to start. Integrated spasticity management needs to start earlier in the young and be offered to adults with cerebral palsy.

The universal problem in any neurologic injury is muscle weakness, but it is harder to recognize and treat in a small child than it is in an adult. But if you do strengthen a child's muscles after a brain injury, it can help the child gain the ability to move normally. Strengthening protocols in children have been tested and the evidence is in.[3] It works.

If maladaptive movements are already established, the same treatments may still be applied. They are likely to be more effective if therapists integrate some of the strategies employed by professional coaches. Coaches know about habits; they're experts at replacing bad ones with good. They focus on drills that work around the maladaptive pattern of movement. They use intensives—focused, sustained practice—to build new neural pathways, to change not just the way the muscles move but also the brain that controls movement. Children, especially teens experiencing their second growth spurt, are like athletes on steroids: their brain is growing along with the rest of their body, making them perfect candidates for this kind of treatment.

Some therapists and doctors are reluctant to use technological devices to assist them in their work with children. They know what they can accomplish with patience and their hands and, like the rest of us, they tend to stick with what they know. But technology, appropriately applied, can bring about magical transformations. Properly fitted braces and AFOs are indispensable where alignment has become an issue. Ditto supportive garments, such as TheraTogs, which can help even small children dealing with weakness, alignment, and balance issues. Threshold electrical stimulation is no longer available, which is a pity, because it has its uses. EMG bio-feedback and EMG-triggered stimulation are available and can make the therapist's job both easier and more effective. Adult patients with many different neurologic problems are offered these treatments.[4] At a minimum, children and teens deserve the same opportunity, like Lisa, to discover what their body actually can do.

Constraint-Induced Movement Therapy has been proven in at least twenty randomized controlled trials. Like many other treatments that have been seen to work in research studies, CIMT is more commonly used for adults recovering from stroke than in children with a similar type of brain injury. It should have a place in every therapist's toolbox.

If some of us in the medical profession have been slow to exploit neuroplasticity's potential, others have not hesitated. Surgeons like Bruce Hendrick, who were among the pioneers performing hemispherectomies, were acting on the idea when I, and a great many like me, had no notion of their achievements. Others, like T.S. Park in St. Louis who refined selective dorsal rhizotomy, and Jim Gage and the surgeons at the Gillette Children's Hospital in Minneapolis–St. Paul who refined Single-Event MultiLevel Surgery, demonstrated conclusively that there are effective interventions to restore body alignment and reduce spasticity. The doctors and scientists who made inventive use of Botox and Baclofen pumps to radically change the outlook for children with CP were change artists as well. Progress is the product of developments on many fronts.

While our hope for the future depends upon preventing some and diagnosing and treating other infants with brain damage as early as possible, the condition affects adults too. It is an appalling situation when a man in his forties, who is clearly experiencing the long-term effects of unbalanced movement stemming from CP, is turned away from the centres ostensibly intended to treat the condition. The same therapies that work for children work for adults as well.

Perhaps the most important point that I have learned is that every case is different. The nature and severity of dysfunction depend upon the kind of injury the child sustained, when it happened, and how much damage it did. There is no single therapeutic regime that can be applied in every case. The doctors, parents, and therapists who achieve the best results are open-minded, eclectic, and imaginative. Their treatment plans reflect the unique situation of each individual.

And sometimes the therapies that are effective are shockingly simple. Water exercise (with a Wet Vest) can achieve wonders. Yoga, martial arts, and Pilates can be good for strength and balance. Music may draw on parts of the brain that are otherwise unused and undamaged. Visual signals—coloured masking tape—can have a surprising, positive effect. And look what Suzanne Davis Bombria achieved with bungee cords and a helium-filled balloon!

To use these therapies to help children with cerebral palsy get better, it will take a systemic change. Still today, access to proven therapies is limited, both by institutional preferences and by insurance companies. School-based therapy, available by legislation to all children with special needs, is limited to addressing only educational-based objectives—not to improving motor function. For example, if a child needs to move more rapidly from class to class, a wheelchair is provided. There is no time or funding devoted to teaching him to walk faster. Once he is in a chair, there is little hope of any further motor improvement.

To achieve the systemic change that will offer real hope to young people with CP, we need to change our society's attitude to early brain and nerve injury. On a recent trip to the Shepherd Center in Atlanta, Georgia, I was struck by the difference between traditional pediatric therapy for children with cerebral palsy and brachial plexus injury and the neurorehabilitation offered to adults. The first and most striking difference was that in the adult population, cure is an accepted goal. All the professionals I met had a clear understanding that there were differences in the severity of the neurologic injury, patient to patient, and obviously some were going to have a much better outcome than others. I saw no evidence of false hope, but rather a lot of enthusiasm and interaction between the research and clinical groups who shared the same goal of complete recovery for some, and a best possible outcome for the rest.

Contrast this with the position taken by the authors of a textbook on cerebral palsy published in 2012: "While there may be *no hope for a cure* … there is much that can be done to enhance child and family development and well-being."[5]

Why is the possibility of a cure rejected with such finality? The resigned, negative certainty of this pronouncement reflects the same fixed mindset (to use Carol Dweck's term) that leads to a well-meaning but passive focus on the child with cerebral palsy's "quality of life" rather than a growth mindset that entertains the possibility of turning around his dysfunctional behaviour. It stems from belief in a paradigm whose time is past.

Everyone, in both pediatric and adult rehabilitation, wants the best possible outcome for their patients. Yet a goal that falls short of complete recovery is dispiriting. No coach tells a runner who's training for a hundred-metre race that it's fine if she pulls out after twenty-five metres. No physician treating a youth with a hemiplegic gait should tell him that he's certain to have unbalanced movement for the rest of his life. In both cases, the physician or coach would be saying that it's okay to accept less than your best possible outcome.

The communities of people affected by other disorders have figured this out. The actor Christopher Reeves was one of a number of men and women who have led a highly visible and successful campaign to make finding a cure the goal of research into spinal cord injury. We're all aware of similar campaigns for breast cancer, autism, muscular dystrophy, and heart disease. No one accuses the people leading these campaigns of being deluded or of spreading false hope. On the contrary, they're admired for their belief in the possibility of a cure. It's an attitude that inspires hope and change.

The Beyond Therapy Program at the Shepherd Center in Atlanta is a tangible demonstration of what can be achieved when healthcare professionals push beyond the barriers of traditional neurorehabilitation. The people I saw on the day I visited had all been discharged from therapy. Some were sent away because they had reached a plateau and no further gains were expected. Others were told that, having attained the functional goals set by their therapy team, they could expect no further improvement. Sound familiar? And yet, at the clinic in Atlanta, they now were achieving a higher level of function! It was inspiring to listen to these patients talk about what they had done. Their long-term goal was to return to their pre-injury status. I have no paranormal powers that would tell me which ones were going to get there, but like athletes in training for Olympic Gold, they had their short-, medium-, and long-range goals to motivate them.

We should be aiming for a cure in the field of pediatric neurorehabilitation as well. Baby brains have more neuro-plasticity than adult brains and we should expect a far greater degree of recovery, and in many cases a cure. Setting a goal of anything less makes no sense to me. I have seen children achieve complete recovery after well-documented early brain or nerve damage. In the vast majority of these cases, I would attribute most of the children's recovery to parents who refused to accept less than a cure as the goal for their child. Not all children will be cured by a change in attitude—but some will, and the rest will benefit from a positive outlook. My goal for children with early brain, nerve, or spinal cord damage is a cure for some and improvement for all. This is real hope for a better future and it is a change that together we can achieve.

acknowledgments

I would like to thank my publisher, Sarah Scott, who added her passion to mine in bringing this book to life. From the outset, she saw the need for a book and was a strong advocate, introducing me to her excellent publishing team. Thanks to Jonathan Webb, whose comprehensive structural edit gave bones to the material and who, along with Sarah, showed me how best to tell my story. Special thanks to the excellent production team led by Tracy Bordian that included designer and formatter Kyle Gell, copy editor Marcia Gallego, proofreader Heather Sangster/Strong Finish Editorial Design, and indexer Wendy Thomas. Thanks also to Margie Miller for a cover design that captures the essence of *The Boy Who Could Run But Not Walk*.

This book would not have been possible without the work of an army of basic and applied neuroscientists, physicians, surgeons, psychologists, and biomedical engineers pushing the boundaries of traditional thinking about the human brain. The neuroplasticity revolution is now well underway as a result of their collective endeavors.

Over 30 years ago, I attended an inspirational talk by neuroscientist Michael Merzenich at a Society for Neuroscience meeting in which he demonstrated the power of activity dependent neuroplasticity. Years after, Norman Doidge brought his work, along with many of the other intellectual outliers that have shaped our present understanding of the brain, to the attention of the general public. In different ways, they both have played a major part in shaping my theories of baby brain neuroplasticity. I thank them.

A special thank you to another, smaller army of physicians, surgeons, therapists, and nurses who have contributed to my understanding of how the baby brain recovers from early injury. I will be forever indebted to the families and individuals who took a leap of faith, trusted that I knew what I was doing, and have shared their stories in this book. Christine Rouse, an adult with choreoathetosis, took the biggest leap of faith and proved that it truly is never too late to make new habits to replace the old.

I would also like to thank my critics and detractors for their help in honing my theories. As Thomas Kuhn would say, they too are an important part of a scientific revolution.

Finally, thank you to my assistant, Wing Sei Lam, for over 16 years of listening to my stories and organizing my life so well, and to Paul Bonish for his excellent technical support. A book for the public has to reach the public, and I am also indebted to Yvonne Hunter, Katrina Weidknecht, and Debby de Groot for their wisdom and help in achieving this goal.

glossary

Activity-Dependent Neuroplasticity: The ability of the brain to change in response to what input it receives on a day-to-day basis. Skill in any activity depends on repetition. After a neurologic loss, the brain may be able to rewire to account for the injury with purposeful, intensive practice.

Amblyopia, or Lazy Eye: A medical term that describes unilateral visual inattention. The eye looks normal, but the brain is actively ignoring the visual input.

Ankle Foot Orthoses (AFOs): A brace, often made of plastic, worn on the lower leg and foot to support the ankle and to hold the foot and ankle in correct position. This is the most commonly used brace in children with cerebral palsy.

Anomalies: Something that deviates from what is standard, normal, or expected.

Apgar Score: Stands for Appearance (skin colour), Pulse (heart rate), Grimace (reflex responsiveness), Activity (muscle tone), and Respiration (breathing rate and effort). It is a quick assessment of the baby's condition with a three-point scale of 0, 1, or 2 at one, five, and ten minutes after birth. The maximum score is 10.

Asphyxia: A total brain and body injury caused by decreased oxygen and excess carbon dioxide in the blood. In newborn babies it is most often seen following a difficult delivery process and/or lung diseases.

Ataxia: Considered the rarest form of cerebral palsy, affecting balance and fine motor skills. Intelligence is usually unaffected.

Athetosis: A movement disorder that causes a continuous stream of slow, flowing, writhing involuntary movements. Formerly the most common form of cerebral palsy, it now affects less than 10 percent of children with cerebral palsy. Intelligence is usually unaffected, but orofacial and speech impairments are common.

Basal Ganglia, or Basal Nuclei: Multiple subcortical nuclei located at the base of the forebrain. The basal ganglia interact widely with other parts of the brain in the control of voluntary motor movements, procedural learning, eye movements, cognition, and emotion. Injury to them in the newborn infant produces athetosis and/or choreoathetosis.

Bayley Scales of Infant Development (BSID-III is the current version): A standard series of measurements used to assess overall development of infants and toddlers age zero to three years.

Botulinum Toxin (BTX): A neurotoxic protein produced by the bacterium *Clostridium botulinum* and related species. It is used for medical, cosmetic, and research use. Botulinum type A and botulinum type B are the trade names of this drug in use for children with cerebral palsy.

Brachial Plexus Injury (BPI): The brachial plexus is a group of nerve fibres that runs from the spine and through the neck into the arms. In infants a brachial plexus injury can occur in any part of the nerve fibres and can range in severity depending on the location of the injury. One of the most common causes of infant brachial plexus injuries is excessive stretching and force during labour and delivery.

Cerebellum: The cerebellum has an important role in motor control. Although it does not initiate movement, the cerebellum contributes to coordination, precision, and accurate timing. It receives input from sensory systems of the spinal cord and from other parts of the brain, and integrates these inputs to fine-tune motor activity. Cerebellar damage produces disorders in fine movement, equilibrium, posture, and motor learning.

Cerebral Palsy (CP): Cerebral palsy is a generic term that groups together a wide group of disorders that affect a person's ability to move. It encompasses damage to the developing brain during pregnancy, in the perinatal period, or in the first two years of life. Depending upon the site of brain damage, children can have problems with muscle control, coordination, tone (too tight or too floppy), posture, and balance.

Choreoathetosis: Individuals with this type of cerebral palsy have involuntary movements in a combination of chorea and athetosis. Chorea is repetitive, brief, irregular, and rapid involuntary movements.

Cochlear Implant (CI): A surgically implanted electronic device that provides a sense of sound to a person who is profoundly deaf or severely hard of hearing in both ears.

Comorbidity: In medicine, the presence of one or more additional disorders (or diseases) co-occurring with a primary disease or disorder.

Congenital Clubfoot: A range of foot abnormalities present at birth (congenital) in which the baby's foot is twisted out of shape or positioned at a sharp angle to the ankle. Clubfoot occurs in roughly 1 case per 1000 live births in the USA.

Cortical Visual Impairment (CVI): A form of visual impairment that is caused by a brain problem rather than an eye problem.

Corticospinal System: The principal brain system for controlling movement. It matures over a prolonged period and is modified by experience (skill development).

Dichoptic: A term that describes a research method where each eye is presented with a different visual field, forcing the eyes to work independently.

Diplegia: Diplegic cerebral palsy is a form of cerebral palsy that primarily affects motor control of the legs. The majority of children have spastic (tight) leg muscles, although a few have low tone without spasticity. Diplegia is the most common form of cerebral palsy in babies born early. Most children have normal intelligence, although learning disabilities (a common problem in premature babies) may cause some delay in the early years.

Disuse Muscle Atrophy: Muscles that are not used rapidly waste away and lose strength. Children and adults with neurologic problems all have some degree of disuse muscle atrophy in addition to their neurologic problem, which contributes to their level of impairment.

Dyskinesia: A category of movement disorders that are characterized by involuntary muscle movements and diminished voluntary movements. Dyskinesia can be anything from a slight tremor of the hands to an uncontrollable movement of the upper body or lower extremities. Dyskinetic cerebral palsy includes athetosis, choreoathetosis, and ataxia.

EMG Biofeedback: A technique that picks up small electromyographic (EMG) signals from a target muscle and displays them as a visual and/ or auditory signal. The person with cerebral palsy or brachial plexus injury then learns how to turn the signal up (tightening a weak muscle) or down (relaxing a spastic muscle).

EMG-Triggered Stimulation (ETS): Small electromyographic (EMG) signals are used to trigger a neuromuscular stimulation to increase activation and help strengthen the muscle. It is a form of closed-loop feedback that is effective in rehabilitation of adults with stroke and children with cerebral palsy, combining neuromuscular electrical stimulation (NMES) with EMG biofeedback in one device.

Facilitated Brain, or Neural Network: *Neurons that fire together wire together*, a phrase attributed to D.O. Hebb, is the underlying process of creating a habit in the brain. Facilitated networks or circuits fire more readily and transmit their neural impulses faster.

Fontanel, or Soft Spot: An anatomical feature of the infant human skull comprising the soft membranous gaps (sutures) between the cranial bones that make up the skull of a fetus or an infant. They are quite large in premature infants.

Functional Magnetic Resonance Imaging (fMRI): A specialized brain scan that measures brain activity by detecting changes associated with blood flow. When an area of the brain is in use, blood flow to that region increases.

Germinal Matrix (also known as Subependymal Capillary Bed): A highly cellular and vascularized region in the brain from which cells migrate out during brain development. The germinal matrix is the source of both neurons and glial cells and is most active between eight and thirty-two to thirty-four weeks gestation. It is the most common source of both a localized and/or an intraventricular hemorrhage.

Gross Motor Function Measure (GMFM): A clinical tool to evaluate gross motor function in children with cerebral palsy from lying and rolling up to walking, running, and jumping skills. There are two versions of the GMFM: the original eighty-eight-item measure (GMFM-88) and the more recent sixty-six-item GMFM (GMFM-66). This test measures the child's *usual* behaviour.

Hemidecortication: The surgical removal of one half of the cortex of the brain in young rats.

Hemiplegia: A form of cerebral palsy that affects the arm and leg on one side of the body. Babies born at term with hemiplegia may also experience speech problems and are prone to more seizures than babies with other forms of cerebral palsy.

Hemispherectomy: A surgical procedure where one cerebral hemisphere (half of the brain) is removed or disabled. This procedure is used to treat a variety of seizure disorders where the source of the epilepsy is localized to a hemisphere of the brain.

Hip Flexors: A group of muscles that includes the iliopsoas, the thigh muscles (rectus femoris, sartorius, and tensor fasciae latae), and the inner thigh muscles (adductor longus and brevis, pectineus, and gracilis). These muscles tend to tighten and shorten with growth in children with spastic cerebral palsy.

Hydrocephalus: Cerebrospinal fluid (CSF) is a clear fluid that normally circulates through and surrounds the brain and spinal cord. If this is blocked, excessive accumulation of CSF results in an abnormal widening of the ventricles, creating harmful pressure on the tissues of the brain. The head of a baby is able to compensate to some degree by separating the sutures of the skull to relieve pressure.

Iatrogenic: An adverse medical or surgical complication arising from a treatment or procedure or a drug interaction. Some are expected side effects and some are due to misadventure.

Intrathecal Baclofen Pump (ITB): An implanted device that delivers the drug Baclofen directly to the fluid surrounding the spinal cord. Baclofen decreases spasticity by damping down hyperactive reflexes and excessive muscle tone. It is used in children with cerebral palsy, most commonly in children with severe spastic quadriplegia.

Intraventricular Hemorrhage (IVH): Bleeding into the central ventricles of the brain. It often occurs in the distressed baby in the first few days of life in premature infants. This bleeding originates in the subependymal germinal matrix, a vulnerable area in the developing brain that matures and involutes by thirty-two to thirty-four weeks gestational age. It is rarely seen in a full-term infant.

Ischemia: A restriction in blood supply to tissues, causing a shortage of oxygen and glucose needed for cellular metabolism (to keep tissue alive).

Ischemic Stroke: Ischemic strokes (clots) occur as a result of an obstruction within a blood vessel supplying blood to the brain, which usually affects one side of the brain.

Isolette: An enclosed neonatal bed that provides a controlled heat, humidity, and oxygen microenvironment for the isolation and care of premature and low birth-weight newborns.

Kernicterus: A rare neurologic condition that occurs in some newborns with severe jaundice (very high levels of bilirubin). This can lead to brain damage and hearing loss.

Kinesiology, or Human Kinetics: The study of human movement with an emphasis on biomechanics of movement, strength and conditioning, sport psychology, methods of neurologic rehabilitation, and sport and exercise.

Maladaptive: Behaviour or actions that interfere with activities of daily living.

Median Nerve Damage: Injury of the median nerve at the elbow causes motor and sensory deficits affecting the thumb and index finger of the hand.

Menarche: The first menstrual cycle, or first menstrual bleeding, in female humans.

Meningitis: An inflammation of the membranes (meninges) surrounding the brain and spinal cord. It may be caused by a bacterial, viral, or fungal infection.

Metronome: A device that produces regular, evenly spaced sounds (beats, clicks). The number of beats per minute can be set.

Motor Cortex: A region of the cerebral cortex involved in the planning, control, and execution of voluntary movements. It is the area of the brain that directs the corticospinal system, which includes the cortex, the brainstem nuclei, the cerebellum, the spinal cord, and the peripheral motor nerves that terminate at the muscles.

Nada Chair: A flexible sling that provides back support in the proper anatomical alignment. The most common uses are for low back pain.

Neonatology: A sub-specialty of pediatrics that consists of the medical care of distressed newborn infants. It is a hospital-based practice in neonatal intensive care units (NICU).

Neural Circuits: Interconnected neurons that regulate their activity with both positive and negative feedback loops. Large groups of neural circuits may form into a neural network.

Neuroblast: An immature dividing cell that will develop into a neuron (nerve cell) often after a migration phase.

Neurogenesis: New neurons (brain cells) are generated from neural stem cells and progenitor cells. Neurogenesis is most active during prenatal development, the first four to six years, and again for four to six years during the pubertal growth spurt.

Neuromuscular Electrical Stimulation (NMES): Also known as electrical muscle stimulation (EMS), a method of eliciting an active muscle contraction by electric impulses to the skin. NMES is used as a strength-training tool for both injured athletes and children with cerebral palsy. It uses a strong current level to depolarize the muscle and it can be uncomfortable.

Neurons (Nerve Cells): These brain cells are the core components of the brain and spinal cord of the central nervous system, and of the ganglia of the peripheral nervous system. There are many specialized types of neurons that perform different functions.

Neuro-ophthalmologist: Eye doctors who specialize in visual problems caused by injury to the brain, not the eye. This is a sub-specialty of both neurology and ophthalmology, requiring specialized training and expertise in problems of the eye, brain, nerves, and muscles.

Neuropathologist: A pathologist who specializes in the diagnosis of diseases of the brain and nervous system by gross and microscopic examination of the tissue.

Neuroplasticity: Also known as brain plasticity, a generic term that describes lasting change to the brain throughout life. Scientists now understand that human brains can grow new cells, repair damage, wire new connections, and reallocate brain real estate to compensate for brain damage.

Neurorehabilitation: A process with the goal of aiding recovery from a nervous system injury and to minimize and/or compensate for any functional alterations resulting from it.

Neuropsychology: A field of neuroscience concerned with the diagnosis and treatment of behavioural and cognitive effects of neurologic disorders. This field encompasses brain/mind interfaces.

OBS Charts: A short-form term for charts of pregnant women seen in an obstetrical clinic.

Obsessive-Compulsive Disorder (OCD): A mental disorder in which a person has uncontrollable, repetitive, intrusive thoughts and behaviours, such as the need to clean excessively, check on things, and perform certain routines.

Occipital Lobes of the Brain: Located at the rear portion of the skull, behind the parietal and temporal lobes. This area is the primary visual cortex where visual inputs are processed.

Occupational Therapy (OT): Licensed professionals who participate in the treatment of children with cerebral palsy, working in conjunction with physical therapists and speech therapists. In pediatrics, their focus is primarily on the rehabilitation of the upper trunk, arms, and hands.

Outliers: In classic statistics, an observation point that is distant from other observations. In medicine, a person or thing differing from all other members of a particular group. Outliers complicate our ability to determine an accurate prognosis for the individual child and are often ignored as "a lucky exception to the rule." See also *anomalies*.

Paradigm: A distinct set of concepts, including theories, research methods and postulates that become a standard for what constitutes legitimate science. Paradigms change with new knowledge. Thomas Kuhn popularized the term "paradigm shift" to express a new way of thinking about an old problem.

Patterning: A controversial physical therapy approach based on the principle that children with cerebral palsy should be taught motor skills in the same sequence in which they develop in normal children. Therapists begin by teaching a child elementary movements such as crawling—regardless of age—before moving on to walking skills.

Peabody Developmental Motor Scales (PDMS-2): An early childhood motor development assessment of gross and fine motor skills from birth through five years of age.

Perinatal Period: Starts at the twenty-third to twenty-fourth week of gestation and ends roughly four weeks after birth.

Periventricular Leukomalacia (PVL): A particular type of brain damage most commonly seen in babies born prematurely less than thirty-four weeks of gestation. It is found in the white matter of the brain and primarily affects the control of the legs, although extensive lesions may also affect the arms. It is strongly associated with spastic diplegia.

Physiatrist, or Physical Medicine and Rehabilitation (PM&R) Physicians: Medical specialists treating conditions affecting the brain, spinal cord, nerves, bones, joints, ligaments, muscles, and tendons. Some of these physicians have also specialized in pediatrics and work with children with brain or nerve injuries.

Physical Therapist (PT): Pediatric PTs are licensed healthcare professionals who provide care for children in a variety of settings, including hospitals, private practices, outpatient clinics, schools, and sports and fitness facilities. Their focus in children with cerebral palsy is to facilitate the child learning how to move, muscle strengthening, and fitness. There is very little focus on pediatric neuromotor problems in the primary university degree, with most learning about CP occurring in on-the-job training and continuing education programs.

Post-Polio Syndrome: Many years after recovering from polio, survivors may experience gradual new weakening in muscles that were previously affected by the polio infection. Some individuals experience only minor symptoms while others develop visible muscle weakness and atrophy.

Prefrontal Lobes of the Cortex: The prefrontal cortex (PFC) is located in the very front of the brain, just behind the forehead. It is the latest-maturing part of the brain. This area regulates a wide group of executive functions, including abstract thinking, social control, consciousness, general intelligence, and personality.

Proprioceptive System: A system that provides sensory inputs concerning the body's position in space. The sense of proprioception is affected in most children with cerebral palsy, particularly in those with spastic quadriplegia, athetosis, choreoathetosis, and ataxia.

Quadriplegia: A form of cerebral palsy that affects all four limbs and is the most severe form. The child may have spasticity with tight muscles or one of the dyskinetic forms: athetosis, choreoathetosis, or ataxia. The exact expression of this topography is determined by the site and extent of brain damage.

Rasmussen's Encephalitis: Also known as chronic focal encephalitis (CFE). A rare inflammatory neurologic disease characterized by frequent and severe seizures, loss of motor skills and speech, hemiparesis (paralysis on one side of the body), encephalitis (inflammation of the brain), and dementia. The illness affects a single cerebral hemisphere and generally occurs in children under the age of fifteen.

Retrolental Fibroplasia: An abnormal proliferation of fibrous tissue immediately behind the lens of the eye, leading to blindness. It occurs primarily in babies born prematurely.

Rhesus Incompatibility: Develops when the mother is Rh-negative and the infant is Rh-positive. This problem has become less common since a preventative treatment (RhoGHAM) is now routinely used to prevent it when the mother's blood type is Rh-negative.

Sacroiliac (SI) Joint: The joint in the bony pelvis between the sacrum and the ilium of the pelvis, which are joined by strong ligaments. The sacrum supports the spine and is supported in turn by an ilium on each side.

Scattergram, or Scatter Plot: Graphic representation of a data set of points in two planes. It rapidly identifies outliers that are distant from the bulk of the data points.

Selection Bias: A non-random selection of study participants.

Selective Dorsal Rhizotomy (SDR): A neurosurgical procedure that involves cutting a proportion of the sensory nerve fibres that comes from the spastic muscles at the level of the spinal cord. This reduces sensory feedback (messages) from the muscle, resulting in less spasticity.

Somatosensory System: The parts of the brain that allow the perception of touch, pressure, pain, temperature, position, movement, and vibration, which arise from the muscles, joints, skin, and fascia.

Spasticity: After damage to the brain or spinal motor system, excess, involuntary contraction of some muscles causes stiffness or tightness of the muscles that may interfere with normal hand use, speech, and/or gait. The areas of the body that are affected are determined by the areas of the brain that are damaged. In children, spasticity and body growth interact to worsen the condition.

Stroke: A sudden loss of brain function caused by the interruption of flow of blood to the brain (ischemic stroke) or the rupture of blood vessels in the brain (hemorrhagic stroke). The interruption of blood flow or the rupture of blood vessels causes brain cells (neurons) in the affected area to die. The effects of a stroke depend on where the brain was injured, as well as how much damage occurred. The motor effects of a one-sided stroke are similar to hemiplegia in a child.

Sturge-Weber Syndrome, or Sturge-Weber-Dimitri Syndrome: A congenital, non-familial disorder of unknown incidence and cause. It is characterized by a congenital facial birthmark and neurologic abnormalities, including severe seizures.

Synapses: A structure that permits a neuron (or nerve cell) to pass an electrical or chemical signal to another neuron. A synaptic junction is a similar structure that passes a chemical signal to another cell, such as the communication between a nerve cell and a muscle cell.

Therapeutic Orphans: A term coined in 1968 by H. Shirkey for the lack of studies about the safety, dosing, and efficacy of drugs used in children that have been approved for adults. I use it to describe a situation where therapies and interventions shown to be effective in adult neurologic problems are not studied or made available to children.

Threshold Electrical Stimulation (TES): Surface electrical stimulation used overnight during sleep at a very low intensity. This level of stimulation, just at the sensory level, is a sub-contraction level that does not make the muscle contract. Children have described the sensation as "butterfly kisses."

Tracheotomy: A surgical procedure to open a direct airway through an incision in the trachea (windpipe). In infants needing prolonged mechanical ventilation, it is used to bypass the mouth, allowing the infant to eat and later to talk with a modified tracheostomy attachment called a talking tracheostomy.

Transient Dystonia: Various abnormalities of muscle tone seen in mainly premature infants in the first one to two years of life. Muscle tone may be decreased (hypotonia) or increased (hypertonia). If these abnormalities persist to the two-year mark, the diagnosis is changed to cerebral palsy. If it resolves, it is considered to be transient dystonia.

Ventilator: A machine designed to mechanically breathe for a patient who is unable to breathe effectively.

Vestibular System: The sensory system for balance and spatial orientation. It sends signals to the muscles that control eye movements and to the muscles that keep the body upright.

Wet Vest: A snug-fitting vest with flotation panels and a thermal layer that is used by athletes and rehabilitation patients to provide support while exercising in deep water. It provides an ideal "out-of-gravity" training method for children and adults with cerebral palsy.

introduction

1. Johannes Borgstein and Caroline Grootendorst, "Half a Brain," *The Lancet* 359, no. 9305 (2002): 473. There is a more complete discussion of hemispherectomy in both animals and children in Chapter 2.

2. Roger Lewin, "Is Your Brain Really Necessary?" *Science* 210, no. 12 (1980): 1232–34.

3. Thomas S. Kuhn, *The Structure of Scientific Revolutions* (Chicago: University of Chicago Press, 1962). A fiftieth anniversary edition of this book, with a new introductory essay by Ian Hacking, was published in 2012.

4. "NINDS Cerebral Palsy Information Page," National Institute of Neurological Disorders and Stroke, accessed Jan. 9, 2016, http://www.ninds.nih.gov/disorders/cerebral_palsy/cerebral _palsy.htm. Italics added.

one

1. Iona Novak, "Evidence-Based Diagnosis, Health Care, and Rehabilitation for Children with Cerebral Palsy," *Journal of Child Neurology* 29 (2014): 1141–56.

2. Norman Doidge, *The Brain That Changes Itself* (New York: Penguin Books, 2007). This book changed the public and professional understanding of neuroplasticity and has led to major improvements in many areas of adult neurology. It is a highly recommended read for anyone interested in the human brain.

3. Michael Merzenich, *Soft-Wired* (San Francisco: Parnassus, 2013), 14–17. The book provides a fascinating description of the life's work of a true pioneer in the field of neuroplasticity.

two

1. "NINDS Cerebral Palsy Information Page," accessed Jan. 9, 2016. Italics added.

2. "NINDS Stroke Information Page," National Institute of Neurological Disorders and Stroke, last modified Dec. 11, 2015, http://www.ninds.nih.gov/disorders/stroke/stroke.htm. Italics added.

3. D.O. Hebb, *The Organization of Behaviour: A Neuropsychological Theory* (New York: John Wiley & Sons, 1949), 287. A fiftieth anniversary edition of this book was published by Psychology Press in 2002.

4. Ibid., 62.

5. R. Melzack and P.D. Wall, "Pain Mechanisms: A New Theory," *Science* 150 (1965): 971–79.

6. Stephen McMahon, Martin Koltzenburg, Irene Tracey, and Dennis C. Turk, *Wall and Melzack's Textbook of Pain*, 6th ed. (Philadelphia: Elsevier/Saunders, 2013).

7. G. Koren, W. Butt, H. Chinyanga, S. Soldin, Y.-K. Tan, and K.E. Pape, "Postoperative Morphine Infusion in Newborn Infants: Assessment of Disposition Characteristics and Safety," *Journal of Pediatrics* 197 (1985): 963–70.

8. Carlo V. Bellieni and C. Celeste Johnston, "Analgesia, Nil or Placebo to Babies, in Trials That Test New Analgesic Treatments for Procedural Pain," *Acta Paediatrica* 105 (2015): 129–36.

9. Iona Novak, "Evidence-Based Diagnosis, Health Care, and Rehabilitation for Children with Cerebral Palsy," *Journal of Child Neurology* 29 (2014): 1141–56.

10. K. Magee, J. Basinska, B. Quarrington, and H.C. Stancer, "Blindness and Menarche," *Life Sciences* 9 (1970): Part 1, 7–12.

11. W. Silverman, "The Lesson of Retrolental Fibroplasia," *Scientific American* 236 (1977): 100–107.

12. BOOST II, "Oxygen Saturation and Outcomes in Preterm Infants," *New England Journal of Medicine* 368 (2013): 2094–104.

13. M.O. Bakheit, "Optimising the Methods of Evaluation of the Effectiveness of Botulinum Toxin Treatment of Post-Stroke Muscle Spasticity," *Journal of Neurology, Neurosurgery and Psychiatry* 75 (2004): 665–66.

14. Paul R. Swyer, "Babies: The Fight for Intact Survival at the Hospital for Sick Children, 1875–2000: A Personal View" (Toronto: Privately printed, circa 2005), 23–24.

15. Ibid., 52.

three

1. Adele Diamond, "Close Interrelation of Motor Development and Cognitive Development and of the Cerebellum and Prefrontal Cortex," *Child Development* 71 (2000): 44–56.

2. Maren C. Kiessling et al., "Cerebellar Granule Cells Are Generated Postnatally in Humans," *Brain Structure and Function* 219 (2014): 1271–86.

3. Joseph J. Volpe, "Neonatal Periventricular Hemorrhage: Past, Present, and Future," *Journal of Pediatrics* 92 (1978): 693–96.

4. G. Hambleton and J.S. Wigglesworth, "Origin of Intraventricular Haemorrhage in the Preterm Infant," *Archives of Disease in Childhood* 51 (1976): 651.

5. Karen E. Pape and Jonathan S. Wigglesworth, *Haemorrhage, Ischaemia and the Perinatal Brain* (London: William Heinemann, 1979), 141.

6. Ibid., 120.

7. Dawna Armstrong and Margaret Norman, "Periventricular Leucomalacia in Neonates," *Archives of Disease in Childhood* 49 (1974): 367–75.

8. J.S. Wigglesworth and K.E. Pape, "An Integrated Model for Hae-morrhagic and Ischaemic Lesions in the Newborn Brain," *Journal of Early Human Development* 2 (1978): 179–99; J.S. Wigglesworth and K.E. Pape, "Pathophysiology of Intracranial Haemorrhage in the Newborn," *Journal of Perinatal Medicine* 8 (1980): 119–33.

9. K.E. Pape et al., "Ultrasound Detection of Brain Damage in Preterm Infants," *Lancet* 313 (1979): 1261–64.

10. A.P. Lipscombe et al., "Ultrasound Scanning of Brain through the Anterior Fontanelle of Newborn Infants," *Lancet* 314 (1979): 39.

11. Harold Hoffman et al., "Hemispherectomy for Sturge-Weber Syndrome," *Child's Brain* 5 (1979): 233–48.

12. Ibid.

13. Pape and Wigglesworth, *Haemorrhage*, 166–74.

14. Bryan Kolb and Robin Gibb, "Brain Plasticity and Behaviour in the Developing Brain," *Journal of the Canadian Academy of Child and Adolescent Psychiatry,* 20 (2011): 265–76.

15. Mark Burke et al., "Adaptive Neuroplastic Responses in Early and Late Hemispherectomized Monkeys," *Neural Plasticity* 2012. doi:10.1155/2012/852423.

16. Thomas S. Kuhn, *The Structure of Scientific Revolutions*, 4th ed. (Chicago: University of Chicago Press, 2012), 23–34.

17. J.S. Wigglesworth, "Plasticity of the Developing Brain," in *Peri-natal Brain Lesions*, ed. K.E. Pape and J.S. Wigglesworth. Con-temporary Issues in Foetal and Neonatal Medicine (London: Blackwell Science, 1989), 253–69.

18. Pape and Wigglesworth, *Perinatal Brain Lesions*.

four

1. S. Shah et al., "Screening with MRI for Accurate and Rapid Stroke Treatment: SMART," *Neurology* 84 (2015): 2438–44.

2. Karin B. Nelson and Jonas H. Ellenberg, "Apgar Scores as Predictors of Chronic Neurologic Disability," *Pediatrics* 68 (1981): 36–44.

3. Karen B. Nelson and Jonas H. Ellenberg, "Children Who 'Outgrew' Cerebral Palsy," *Pediatrics* 69 (1982): 529–34, 535.

4. Lu Ann Papile et al., "Incidence and Evolution of Subependymal and Intraventricular Hemorrhage: A Study of Infants with Birth Weight Less than 1,500g," *Journal of Pediatrics* 92 (1978): 529–34.

5. Karen E. Pape, "Etiology and Pathogenesis of Intraventricular Hemorrhage in Newborns," *Pediatrics* 84 (1989): 382–85, 383.

6. Papile et al., "Incidence and Evolution."

7. Lu-Ann Papile et al., "Relationship of Cerebral Intraventricular Hemorrhage and Early Childhood Neurologic Handicaps," *Journal of Pediatrics* 103 (1983): 273–77.

8. Papile et al., "Incidence and Evolution," 529.

9. Joseph J. Volpe, "Neonatal Periventricular Hemorrhage: Past, Present, and Future," *Journal of Pediatrics* 92 (1978): 694. Italics added.

10. Annemieke Brouwer et al., "Neurodevelopmental Outcome of Preterm Infants with Severe Intraventricular Hemorrhage and Therapy for Post-Hemorrhagic Ventricular Dilatation," *Journal of Pediatrics* 153 (2008): 648–54.

11. Ibid., 653.

12. "Data and Statistics for Cerebral Palsy," Centers for Disease Control and Prevention, accessed Sept. 16, 2015, http://www.cdc.gov/ncbddd/cp/data.html.

13. Audrius V. Plioplys et al., "Survival Rates among Children with Severe Neurologic Disabilities," *Southern Medical Journal* 91 (1998): 161–72.

14. These two papers from the Cerebral Palsy Alliance of Australia research group give up-to-date prognostic information about children with cerebral palsy, stressing the need for early intervention in the young and more appropriate treatment in the older child and teenager: Sarah McIntyre et al., "Cerebral Palsy—Don't Delay," *Developmental Disabilities Research Reviews* 17 (2011): 114–29; Iona Novak, "Evidence-Based Diagnosis, Health Care, and Rehabilitation for Children with Cerebral Palsy." *Journal of Child Neurology* 29 (2014): 1141–56.

15. "NINDS Cerebral Palsy Information Page," accessed Jan. 9, 2016. Italics added.

five

1. Kuhn, *The Structure of Scientific Revolutions* (1962).

2. Ibid., 24. Italics added.

3. Carol Dweck, *Mindset* (New York: Random House, 2007).

4. Jerome Groopman, *How Doctors Think* (Boston: Houghton Mifflin, 2007).

5. Glen G. Cayler, "Cardiofacial Syndrome: Congenital Heart Disease and Facial Weakness, a Hitherto Unrecognized Association," *Archives of Disease in Childhood* 44 (1969): 69–75.

6. Karen E. Pape and Douglas Pickering, "Asymmetric Crying Facies: An Index of Other Congenital Anomalies," *Journal of Pediatrics* 81 (1972): 21–30.

7. M. Perlman and S.H. Reisner, "Asymmetric Crying Facies and Congenital Anomalies," *Archives of Disease in Childhood* 48 (1973): 627–29.

8. Groopman, *How Doctors Think*, 260.

9. Richard Smith, "Strategies for Coping with Information Overload," *British Medical Journal* 341 (2010): 1281–82.

10. Alan G. Fraser and Frank D. Dunstan, "On the Impossibility of Being Expert," *British Medical Journal* 341 (2010): 1314–15.

six

1. High spinal cord injury is a very rare injury. I had seen only one case before in England, when I was working with Jonathan Wigglesworth. That baby had died at six hours and was only the fourth case ever reported in the English medical literature. J.S. Wigglesworth, "Pathology of Intrapartum and Early Neonatal Death in the Normally Formed Infant," in *Textbook of Fetal and Perinatal Pathology*, ed. J.S. Wigglesworth and D.B. Singer (London: Blackwell Science, 1998), 75–86.

     Years later, my colleague Max Perlman headed an in-depth review of fifteen cases of neonatal high spinal cord injury and found that all of them were associated with a forceps rotation delivery. S.M. Menticoglou et al., "High Cervical Spinal Cord Injury in Neonates Delivered with Forceps: Report of 15 Cases," *Obstetrics and Gynecology* 86 (1995): 589–94.

2. Alex R. Ward and Nataliya Shkuratova, "Russian Electrical Stimulation: The Early Experiments," *Physical Therapy* 82, no. 10 (2002): 1019–30.

3. Karen E. Pape, Susan E. Kirsch, Aharon Galil, Jill E. Boulton, M. Anne White, and Mary Chipman, "Neuromuscular Approach to the Motor Deficits of Cerebral Palsy: A Pilot Study," *Journal of Pediatric Orthopedics* 13 (1993): 628–33.

4. The conventional practice is to run a pilot trial for a new therapy with the most severely affected patients, working on the "chicken soup" principle, meaning that it can't hurt. Equally unscientific is the common practice of running small trials with children with a wide spectrum of severity. To my mind, these practices amount to negative selection bias. There are many techniques that work well in addressing problems of mild to moderate severity that are ineffective in the most severe cases. Testing the most severely involved first did not make sense; neither did including potential non-responders in a small trial where they might lead you to underestimate the effect of the

therapy. TES was not a drug and it wasn't invasive. If the goal was to achieve "normal" function, then it was sensible to start at the mild end of the spectrum.

seven

1. M. Anne White and Karen E. Pape, "The Slump Test," *American Journal of Occupational Therapy* 46 (1992): 271–74.

2. J. Boulton et al., "Reliability of the Peabody Developmental Gross Motor Scale in Children with Cerebral Palsy," *Physical and Occupational Therapy in Pediatrics* 15 (1995): 35–51.

3. "NINDS Cerebral Palsy Information Page," accessed Sept. 9, 2015.

4. Throughout the various medical disciplines, clinical research is facing severe problems of both recruitment of young doctors into the field and funding of their research programs. Although much has been written over the past twenty years, effective solutions are still needed. Leon E. Rosenberg, "The Physician-Scientist: An Essential—and Fragile—Link in the Medical Research Chain," *Journal of Clinical Investigation* 103 (1999): 1621–26; David G. Nathan, "Clinical Research: Perceptions, Reality, and Proposed Solutions," *JAMA* 280 (1998): 1427–31; Nancy S. Sung et al., "Central Challenges Facing the National Clinical Research Enterprise," *JAMA* 289 (2003): 1278–87.

5. It is hard to believe, but for the first twenty or so years of my clinical practice, we all taught that strength training should be avoided in patients with spasticity. Dr. Damiano and her colleagues have shown that purposeful strength training, done correctly with appropriate patients, is an effective intervention. Unfortunately, many CP clinics still do not provide effective strength training. Diane L. Damiano and Mark F. Abel, "Functional Outcomes of Strength Training in Spastic Cerebral Palsy," *Archives of Physical Medicine and Rehabilitation* 79 (1998): 119–25; Diane L. Damiano, Karen Dodd, and Nicholas F. Taylor, "Should

We Be Testing and Training Muscle Strength in Cerebral Palsy?" *Developmental Medicine and Child Neurology* 44 (2002): 68–72.

6. Diane L. Damiano, "Activity, Activity, Activity: Rethinking Our Physical Therapy Approach to Cerebral Palsy," *Physical Therapy* 86 (2006): 1534–40.

7. Sharon Cunningham, "The Magee Clinic," *Current (The Magazine of the Spina Bifida and Hydrocephalus Association of Ontario)* 9 (1990): 1–2.

8. Olga Lechky, "Toronto Clinic Takes New Approach to Neurologic Injury, Damage," *Canadian Medical Association Journal* 148, no. 8 (January 1, 1993): 72–74.

9. The letters quoted were printed under the heading "Toronto Clinic's New Approach," in the letters section of the *Canadian Medical Association Journal* 148, no. 8 (April 15, 1993): 1270, 1272, 1275.

10. "What's Fit to Print?" *Canadian Medical Association Journal* 148, no. 8 (April 15, 1993): 1263.

11. "Toronto Clinic's New Approach," 1275.

12. Karen E. Pape, Susan E. Kirsch, and Joanne M. Bugaesti, "New Therapies in Spastic Cerebral Palsy," *Contemporary Pediatrics* (May/June 1990): 6–13, 6.

13. Paul Steinbok, Ann Reiner, and John R.W. Kestle, "Therapeutic Electrical Stimulation Following Selective Posterior Rhizotomy in Children with Spastic Diplegic Cerebral Palsy: A Randomized Clinical Trial," *Developmental Medicine and Child Neurology* 39 (1997): 515–20.

14. Ibid., 519.

eight

1. Paul Bach-y-Rita et al., "Vision Substitution by Tactile Image Projection," *Nature* 221 (1969): 963–64.

2. Doidge, *The Brain That Changes Itself*, 1–26.

3. Buddy Levy, "The Blind Climber Who 'Sees' with His Tongue," *Discover* (July 2008).

4. Merzenich, *Soft-Wired.*

5. Michael Kenney, "Beat it! Listening to Music Leads to Longer Workouts, U of T Researchers Say," *U of T News*, June 19, 2015, accessed March 1, 2016, http://news.utoronto.ca/beat-it-listening-music-leads-longer-workouts-u-t-researchers-say.

6. Edwin Kiester, Jr., and William Kiester, "Birdbrain Breakthrough," *Smithsonian Magazine*, June 2002, 36–38, http://www.smithsonianmag.com/science-nature/birdbrain-breakthrough-64765165/. This is an interesting read on the attempts of the defenders of the past to discredit the idea of human adult neuroplasticity. Michael Specter, "Rethinking the Brain," *The New Yorker*, July 23, 2001, 42.

7. Oliver Sacks, *Musicophilia* (New York: Random House, 2007), 233–58.

8. Joanne Loewy et al., "The Effects of Music Therapy on Vital Signs, Feeding, and Sleep in Premature Infants," *Pediatrics* 131 (2013): 902–18.

9. Joyce L. Chen et al., "Interactions between Auditory and Dorsal Premotor Cortex during Synchronization to Musical Rhythms," *NeuroImage* 32 (2006): 1771–81.

10. Michael Thaut and Gerald McIntosh, "How Music Helps to Heal the Injured Brain," *Cerebrum*, March 24, 2010, accessed Feb. 4, 2016, http://www.dana.org/Cerebrum/2010/How_Music_Helps_to_Heal_the_Injured_Brain__Therapeutic_Use_Crescendos_Thanks_to_Advances_in_Brain_Science/.

11. Mijin Kim and Concetta M. Tomaino, "Protocol Evaluation for Effective Music Therapy for Persons with Nonfluent Aphasia," *Topics in Stroke Rehabilitation* 15 (2008): 555–69; Gottfried Schlaug et al., "From Singing to Speaking: Why Singing May Lead to Recovery of Expressive Language Function in Patients with Broca's Aphasia," *Music Perception* 25 (2008): 315–23.

12. "100+ Published Research Studies," BrainHQ, Posit Science, accessed Oct. 2, 2015, http://www.brainhq.com/world-class-science/published-research.

13. "Brain Resources," BrainHQ, Posit Science, accessed Oct. 2, 2015, http://www.brainhq.com/brain-resources.

14. Torsten N. Wiesel, "Early Explorations of the Development and Plasticity of the Visual Cortex: A Personal View," *Journal of Neurobiology* 41 (1999): 7–9, 9.

15. Charles D. Gilbert and Torsten N. Wiesel, "Receptive Field Dynamics in Adult Primary Visual Cortex," *Nature* 356 (1992): 150–52.

16. Ibid., 150.

17. "Lazy-Eye Disorder—A Promising Therapeutic Approach," *McGill University News*, April 22, 2013, http://www.mcgill.ca/newsroom/channels/news/lazy-eye-disorder-promising-therapeutic-approach-226011.

18. Jinrong Li et al., "Dichoptic Training Enables the Adult Amblyopic Brain to Learn," *Current Biology* 23 (2013): R308–9.

nine

1. Karen E. Pape, D.L. Armstrong, and P.M. Fitzhardinge, "Peripheral Median Nerve Damage Secondary to Brachial Arterial Blood Gas Sampling," *Journal of Paediatrics* 93 (1978): 852–56.

2. Edward Taub, Gitendra Uswatte, and Rama Pidikiti, "Constraint-Induced Movement Therapy: A New Family of Techniques with Broad Application to Physical Rehabilitation—A Clinical Review," *Journal of Rehabilitation Research and Development* 36, no. 3 (1999): 237–51. This was a similar finding to Michael Merzenich's work with cats, which showed that in the absence of sensory input, the brain map of the affected area shrank away. Use it or lose it! Although the nerves that made movement possible were still intact, the loss of sensation made coordinated movement difficult.

3. Sharon Landesman Ramey et al., *Handbook of Pediatric Constraint-Induced Movement Therapy* (CIMT) (Bethesda, MD: AOTA Press, 2013), 4–5.

4. Taub, Uswatte, and Pidikiti, "Constraint-Induced Movement Therapy." See also Doidge, *The Brain That Changes Itself*, 132–54.

5. Landesman Ramey et al., *Handbook of Pediatric*, 4–5.

6. "Constraint-Induced Therapy (CI Therapy) Taub Therapy Clinic," University of Alabama, School of Medicine, accessed Oct. 6, 2015, http://www.uabmedicine.org/patient-care/treatments/ci-therapy.

7. Edward Taub, "Efficacy of Constraint-Induced Movement Therapy for Children with Cerebral Palsy with Asymmetric Motor Impairment," *Pediatrics* 113 (2004): 305–12.

8. "NINDS Brachial Plexus Injuries Information Page," National Institute of Neurological Disorders and Stroke, accessed Oct. 6, 2015, http://www.ninds.nih.gov/disorders/brachial_plexus/brachial_plexus.htm.

9. Peter M. Waters, "Update on Management of Pediatric Brachial Palsy," *Journal of Pediatric Orthopaedics* B 14 (2005): 233–44.

10. T. Brown et al., "Developmental Apraxia Arising from Neonatal Brachial Plexus Palsy," *Neurology* 55 (2000): 24–30.

11. J.D. Rollnik et al., "Botulinum Toxin Treatment of Cocontractions after Birth-Related Brachial Plexus Lesions," *Neurology* 55 (2000): 112–14.

12. Michael J. Noetzel and Jonathan R. Wolpaw, "Editorial: Emerging Concepts in the Pathophysiology of Recovery from Neonatal Brachial Plexus Injury," *Neurology* 55 (July 2000): 5–6, 6.

ten

1. Novak, "Evidence-Based Diagnosis."

2. Peter Rosenbaum and Lewis Rosenbaum, *Cerebral Palsy: From Diagnosis to Adult Life* (London: Mac Keith Press, 2012).

3. Brouwer et al., "Neurodevelopmental Outcome."

4. Novak, "Evidence-Based Diagnosis."

5. Rollnik et al., "Botulinum Toxin Treatment."

6. A. Leland Albright, "Baclofen in the Treatment of Cerebral Palsy," *Journal of Child Neurology* 11 (1996): 77–83; Marjanke A. Hoving et al., "Efficacy of Intrathecal Baclofen Therapy in Children with Intractable Spastic Cerebral Palsy: A Randomized Controlled Trial," *European Journal of Paediatric Neurology* 13 (2009): 240–46.

7. Warwick J. Peacock and Loretta A. Staudt, "Spasticity in Cerebral Palsy and the Selective Posterior Rhizotomy Procedure," *Journal of Child Neurology* 5 (1990): 179–85; Nelleke G. Langerak et al., "A Prospective Gait Analysis Study in Patients with Diplegic Cerebral Palsy 20 Years after Selective Dorsal Rhizotomy," *Journal of Neurosurgery: Pediatrics* 1 (2008): 180–86.

8. "About Selective Dorsal Rhizotomy (SDR)," St. Louis Children's Hospital, accessed Oct. 1, 2015, http://www.stlouischildrens .org/our-services/center-cerebral-palsy-spasticity/about- selective-dorsal-rhizotomy-sdr.

9. Novak, "Evidence-Based Diagnosis."

10. "Single Event Multilevel Surgery (SEMLS)," Gillette Children's Specialty Healthcare, accessed Oct. 1, 2015, http://www.gillettechildrens.org/conditions-and-care/ single-event-multilevel-surgery-semls/.

11. Ellen M. Godwin et al., "The Gross Motor Function Classification System for Cerebral Palsy and Single-Event Multilevel Surgery: Is There a Relationship between Level of Function and Intervention over Time?" *Journal of Pediatric Orthopaedics* 29 (2009): 910–15.

eleven

1. McIntyre et al., "Cerebral Palsy—Don't Delay"; Deepa Metgud, V.D. Patil, and S.M. Dhaded, "Predictive Validity of the

Movement Assessment of Infants (MAI) for Six-Month-Old Very Low Birth-Weight Infants," *Journal of Physical Therapy* 3 (2011): 19–23.

2. Iona Novak et al., "A Systematic Review of Interventions for Children with Cerebral Palsy: State of the Evidence," *Developmental Medicine and Child Neurology* 55 (2013): 885–910.

3. Lauran Neergaard, "More Talking, Longer Sentences Help Babies' Brains," *Yahoo! News*, Feb. 14, 2014, accessed Feb. 4, 2016, http://news.yahoo.com/more-talking-longer-sentences-help-babies-39-brains-210215292.html#.

4. For a description of these exercises, see Christine Roman-Lantzy, *Cortical Visual Impairment: An Approach to Assessment and Intervention* (New York: AFB Press, 2007).

5. Novak et al., "A Systematic Review."

6. Tiffany Field, Miguel Diego, and Maria Hernandez-Reif, "Preterm Infant Massage Therapy Research: A Review," *Infant Behavior and Development* 33 (2010): 115–24.

7. Novak, "Evidence-Based Diagnosis."

8. Christina Ragonesi and James C. Galloway, "Short-Term, Early Intensive Power Mobility Training: Case Report of an Infant at Risk for Cerebral Palsy," *Pediatric Physical Therapy* 24 (2012): 141–48; "TEDMED 2014: Cole Galloway," YouTube, https://www.youtube.com/watch?v=PQnPcIGY021.

twelve

1. Novak, "Evidence-Based Diagnosis," 1141.

2. Annoek Louwers et al., "Immediate Effect of a Wrist and Thumb Brace on Bimanual Activities in Children with Hemiplegic Cerebral Palsy," *Developmental Medicine and Child Neurology* 53 (2011): 321–26.

3. Novak et al., "A Systematic Review"; Landesman Ramey et al., *Handbook of Pediatric.*

4. Michael V. Johnston, "Plasticity in the Developing Brain: Implications for Rehabilitation," *Developmental Disabilities Research Reviews* 15 (2009): 94–101.

5. Andrew M. Gordon et al., "Efficacy of a Hand-Arm Bimanual Intensive Therapy (HABIT) in Children with Hemiplegic Cerebral Palsy: A Randomized Control Trial," *Developmental Medicine and Child Neurology* 49 (2007): 830–38; Maya Weinstein et al., "Brain Plasticity Following Intensive Bimanual Therapy in Children with Hemiparesis: Preliminary Evidence," *Neural Plasticity* 2015. doi:10.1155/2015/798481.

6. John Sterba, "Does Horseback Riding Therapy or Therapist-Directed Hippotherapy Rehabilitate Children with Cerebral Palsy?" *Developmental Medicine and Child Neurology* 49 (2007): 68–73.

7. You only need to visit an adaptive sports camp or competition to see how many children are able to run better than they walk. BlazeSports America is the legacy organization of the 1996 Paralympic Games held in Atlanta, Georgia, and a member of the U.S. Olympic Committee Multi-Sport Organizations Council. BlazeSports America provides recreational and competitive adaptive sports experiences and training to a wide variety of children and adults with motor disabilities. Visit http://www.blazesports.org.

   AccesSportAmerica was founded by the family of a young man with cerebral palsy. They provide high-challenge water and land sports for over two thousand children and adults living with challenges/disabilities each year. The sports inspire individuals to train for higher function in AccesSport's year-round training programs. Visit http://www.accessportamerica.org.

thirteen

1. Steven E. Hanna et al., "Stability and Decline in Gross Motor Function among Children and Youth with Cerebral Palsy Aged

2 to 21 Years," *Developmental Medicine and Child Neurology* 51 (2009): 295–302.

2. Robert Palisano et al., "Development and Reliability of a System to Classify Gross Motor Function in Children with Cerebral Palsy," *Developmental Medicine and Child Neurology* 39 (1997): 214–23.

3. P.L. Rosenbaum et al., "Prognosis for Gross Motor Function in Cerebral Palsy: Creation of Motor Development Curves," *JAMA* 2002 (288): 1357–63, 1358.

4. Adrienne Harvey et al., "Current and Future Uses of the Gross Motor Function Classification System," *Developmental Medicine and Child Neurology* 51 (2009): 328–29.

5. Godwin et al., "The Gross Motor Function Classification System."

6. S.E. Hanna et al., "Reference Curves for the Gross Motor Function Measure: Percentiles for Clinical Descriptions and Tracking over Time among Children with Cerebral Palsy," *Physical Therapy* 2008, no. 88: 596–607.

7. Didier Moukoko et al., "Posterior Shoulder Dislocation in Infants with Neonatal Brachial Plexus Palsy," *Journal of Bone and Joint Surgery* 86 (2004): 787–93.

8. Novak et al., "A Systematic Review."

9. Diane Damiano, "Effects of Motor Activity on Brain and Muscle Development in Cerebral Palsy," in *Cerebral Palsy in Infancy: Targeted Activity to Optimize Early Growth and Development*, ed. Roberta Shepherd (Edinburgh: Elsevier Health Sciences, 2013), 196.

fourteen

1. David Strauss et al., "Life Expectancy in Cerebral Palsy: An Update," *Developmental Medicine and Child Neurology* 50 (2008): 487–93.

2. R.H. Gross, C. Scottow, and K. Pape, "Therapeutic Electrical Stimulation for the Treatment of Muscle Weakness Associated with Clubfoot" (Abstract), *Journal of Pediatric Orthopaedics B* 6 (1997): 289.

fifteen

1. McIntyre et al., "Cerebral Palsy—Don't Delay."
2. Eric C. Eichenwald, "Neuroimaging of Extremely Preterm Infants: Perils of Prediction," *Pediatrics* 135 (2015): e176–77.
3. Karen J. Dodd, Nicholas F. Taylor, and Diane L. Damiano, "A Systematic Review of the Effectiveness of Strength-Training Programs for People with Cerebral Palsy," *Archives of Physical Medicine and Rehabilitation* 83 (2002): 1157–64.
4. James H. Cauraugh and Sangbum Kim, "Two Coupled Motor Recovery Protocols Are Better than One: Electromyogram-Triggered Neuromuscular Stimulation and Bilateral Movements," *Stroke* (June 2002): 1589–94; O. Schuhfried et al., "Non-Invasive Neuromuscular Electrical Stimulation in Patients with Central Nervous System Lesions: An Educational Review," *Journal of Rehabilitation Medicine* 44, no. 2 (2012): 99–105, 4.
5. Rosenbaum and Rosenbaum, *Cerebral Palsy*, 112. Italics added.

*T*he goal of this book is to provide information to empower parents of children and adults with an early neurological injury to become informed consumers. The following is a sampling of groups of which I have personal knowledge. I expect this list to grow, and you can find an expanded list on my website at **www.karenpapemd.com**. I am privileged to serve on the Advisory Board of several of these groups; this is indicated by an asterisk (*) next to the name.

Reaching for the Stars* believes that leading-edge pediatric research, increased awareness, and education will lead to new treatments of cerebral palsy, improving the lives of children and their families. It is the largest parent-led group for families affected by cerebral palsy.

Website: reachingforthestars.org

Facebook: facebook.com/ReachingfortheStarsCerebralPalsy

Twitter: twitter.com/reach4stars @Reach4Stars

The Weinberg Family CP Center* is devoted to providing care to patients with cerebral palsy (CP) and their families, as well as guiding care during the transition from childhood to adulthood through a network of adult care specialists knowledgeable about cerebral palsy and related disorders.
Website: columbiaortho.org/specialties/cpcenter
Facebook: facebook.com/WeinbergFamilyCerebralPalsyCenter

The Preemie Family Newsletter* is a resource for families in the NICU and at home. Free to qualified subscribers, each edition is packed with information and resources.
Website: inspire.com/groups/preemie

CP Now improves the lives of people with cerebral palsy and their families by creating educational resources, initiating wellness campaigns, and funding research focussed on addressing the early interferences in brain development that can lead to cerebral palsy.
Website: cpnowfoundation.org
Facebook: facebook.com/CP-Daily-Living-CP-NOW-nonprofit-
199492370144579
Twitter: twitter.com/MyCPNOW

CP Foundation funds research, innovation, and collaboration that changes lives for people with cerebral palsy. Our focus is on the translational research, clinical application, and knowledge transfer that can dramatically change lives—today.
Website: yourcpf.org
Facebook: facebook.com/cerebralpalsyfoundation
Twitter: twitter.com/yourcpf

Three To Be's mission is to support the development of innovative research, therapies, and education for children with neurological disorders and their families.
Website: threetobe.org

Facebook: facebook.com/threetobe

Twitter: twitter.com/threetobe

Cure CP is committed to funding research, studies, trials, and clinical work leading to a cure for cerebral palsy.

Website: curecp.org

Facebook: facebook.com/LetsCureCP

The Children's Hemiplegia and Stroke Association (CHASA) is dedicated to improving the quality of life for children, teens, and young adults who have hemiplegia.

Website: chasa.org

Facebook: facebook.com/Childrens-Hemiplegia-and-Stroke-Association-
   CHASA-153746130096

Twitter: twitter.com/KidsHaveStrokes

Hemikids (part of CHASA) is an email discussion group where parents of infants and children who have hemiplegia or hemiplegic cerebral palsy share information. The parents on Hemi-Kids understand the challenges of parenting a child with mild to moderate hemiplegia.

Website: hemikids.org

Hope for HIE fosters hope in families affected by Hypoxic Ischemic Enceph-alopathy (HIE) through awareness, education, and support.

Website: hopeforhie.org

Facebook: facebook.com/hopeforhie

Twitter: twitter.com/HopeforHIE

The CP Group provides peer support to adults with cerebral palsy who are growing older with the disability. Our members are mentors and activists for youth with cerebral palsy as they transition to adult life.

Website: thecpgroup.org

Email: info@thecpgroup.org

Center for Cerebral Palsy at UCLA strives for excellence in clinical treatment research and education. We are the only interdisciplinary clinic in Southern California that evaluates and treats people with cerebral palsy throughout the lifespan.
Website: uclaccp.org

I am a strong supporter of high-challenge and adapted sports for children and adults with cerebral palsy and other early-acquired brain or nerve problems. Novel challenges stimulate neuroplasticity. The following are two that I know well, but parents should look locally for this type of experience.

BlazeSports America is the legacy organization of the 1996 Paralympic Games held in Atlanta, Georgia, and a member of the United States Olympic Committee Multi Sport Council. BlazeSports America provides recreational and competitive adaptive sports experiences and training to a wide variety of children and adults with motor disabilities.
Website: blazesports.org
Facebook: facebook.com/blazesports
Twitter: twitter.com/blazesports
Email: info@blazesports.org

AccesSportAmerica provides high-challenge water and land sports for children and adults living with challenges/disabilities. Athletes train for higher function in AccesSports' year-round training programs.
Website: accessportamerica.org
Facebook: facebook.com/pages/AccesSportAmerica
Twitter: twitter.com/AccesSport
Instagram: instagram.com/accessport

Children with a hemispherectomy have a range of neurologic causes and outcomes, but intensive therapy can help. They are an important group that often does not have strong local support for research or best therapy after surgery. The following two groups, started by parents, are working to make a difference.

The Hemispherectomy Foundation was founded to provide emotional, financial, and educational support to individuals and their families who have undergone, or will undergo, a hemispherectomy or similar brain surgery.

Website: hemifoundation.homestead.com

Twitter: twitter.com/hemifoundation

Email: Kristi@hemifoundation.org

The Brain Recovery Project Our mission is simple: We help children who have had hemispherectomy surgery reach their full potential.

Website: brainrecoveryproject.org

Facebook: facebook.com/BrainRecoveryProject

Twitter: twitter.com/brainrecoveryp

index

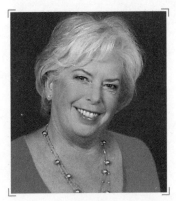

Karen Pape, MD, FRCPC, is a neonatologist and clinical neuroscientist. As a medical innovator, she is challenging the system to raise expectations for babies born with early brain and nerve injury. She was a neonatologist and director of the Neonatal Follow-up Clinic at Toronto's renowned Hospital for Sick Children, with an additional research fellowship in Neonatal Pathology and Ultrasound Brain Scans in London, England. She co-authored a book on baby brain pathology and was instrumental in the development of neonatal ultrasound brain scanning, now used in neonatal intensive care units worldwide. Pape then directed work at the Magee Clinic in Toronto, developing a new, personalized approach to children and adults with early onset brain or nerve damage. She has lectured widely and conducted over 200 training workshops and conferences for parents, therapists, and physicians throughout North America and internationally in 12 countries.

Dr. Pape lives in Toronto, Canada.

www.karenpapemd.com

Library and Archives Canada Cataloguing in Publication data available upon request.

ISBN 978-1-988025-05-6 (hardcover)
ISBN 978-1-988025-06-3 (ebook)

Printed in Canada

TO ORDER:
In Canada:
   Georgetown Publications
   34 Armstrong Avenue, Georgetown, ON L7G 4R9

In the U.S.A.:
   Midpoint Book Sales & Distribution
   27 West 20th Street, Suite 1102, New York, NY 10011

Cover design: Margie Miller
Cover illustration: Eladora, Shutterstock/123RF
Interior design and page layout: Kyle Gell Design

For more information, visit **www.barlowbooks.com**

Barlow Book Publishing Inc.
96 Elm Avenue, Toronto, ON
Canada M4W 1P2

BARLOW BOOKS

THE

BOY

WHO

COULD

RUN

BUT NOT WALK

Understanding Neuroplasticity in the Child's Brain

Karen Pape, MD

with *Jonathan Webb*

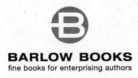

BARLOW BOOKS
fine books for enterprising authors

"Dr. Karen Pape challenges the 'can't do' attitudes surrounding traditional treatment. As parents, we can do no less."

—*Ron Dolenti and Hope Caldwell, parents of twin boys with cerebral palsy*

"Thank you, Dr. Karen Pape, for filling a void for parents who face the vast and intimidating landscape of therapies for children with cerebral palsy. *The Boy Who Could Run But Not Walk* will be my go-to guide for many years to come."

—*Shoshana Hahn-Goldberg, PhD, mother of child with cerebral palsy*

"When my son was 10, the medical field and therapists were unsure and lacking any hope for him to achieve new function or improve. He works out *every day*, played a whole season of sled hockey, and is more comfortable with his body than he has ever been! An absolute *must*-read for parents, physicians, and therapists!"

—*Ruth Grant-Bailey, BSN, RN, mother to Mason Bailey, age 16*

"Like Norman Doidge and Oliver Sacks, Karen Pape challenges medical orthodoxy and breaks new ground. Her work should be required reading for medical students, practicing physicians, physiotherapists, and anyone who works with, coaches, cares for, and loves someone with cerebral palsy."

—*Norah Myers, writer and editor*

"In my late-30s, I was told that I'd never walk unaided again. Dr. Karen Pape had the audacity to believe otherwise. My wish is that this book will encourage doctors not to settle for the status quo, but to look beyond the disabilities they see."

—*Catherine Bell, President, PRIME Impressions, and polio survivor*

"Dr. Karen Pape changes the paradigm 'No hope of a cure' to 'Cure for some and improvement for all,' giving children with brain damage a reason to fight."

—*Lorenzo Beltrame, professional tennis player and coach, awarded*
Coach of the Year and "Doc" Counsilman Science Awards
by the United States Olympic Committee

may preclude further improvements possible in a more mature or recovered nervous system."

"Refreshing and energizing! *The Boy Who Could Run But Not Walk* leads us on a journey not only of hope, but of action."

"Read this book. Dr. Karen Pape offers us the benefit of her remarkable and at times frustrating journey as a neonatologist who would not allow her own unorthodox understanding of the nervous system to be swallowed by conventional medical practices."

"Finally, hope can be passed on to the masses of parents and individuals needing to train smarter and pursue great therapies with success. This book will change lives."

"A solid education in brain injury recovery for the layperson, reminding parents to re-think what they have been told about their child's prognosis."

"The potential for improvement, and even cure, for children with CP and other forms of brain injury appears to be grossly under exploited. *The Boy Who Could Run But Not Walk* offers genuine hope for all parents of at risk and diagnosed children with cerebral palsy."